Marx Joyce
Abbott Hardy Emerson Austen
Defoe Montaigne Cooper Hugo
Melville Machiavelli Chesterton Eliot
Haggard Grimm
Stoker Molière
Christie Maupassant Byron
Wilde Carroll Engels Schiller
Garnett Fitzgerald
Goethe Einstein Hawthorne Kafka
Cotton Dostoyevsky Smith
Baum Kipling Doyle Hall
Leslie Dumas Henry Nietzsche Willis
Flaubert Turgenev Balzac
Stockton Vatsyayana Crane
Burroughs Verne
Curtis Tocqueville Vinci
Homer Widger Tolstoy Gogol Busch
Darwin Whitman
Potter Freud Thoreau Twain Scott Plato Harte
Kant Zola Lawrence
Jowett Stevenson Dickens Burton Hesse
Andersen Cervantes
London Descartes Voltaire
Poe Aristotle Wells
Hale James Hastings Cooke
Bunner Shakespeare
Richter Chambers Irving
Doré da Benedict
Dante Chekhov Shaw Pushkin Alcott
Swift Wodehouse
Newton

tredition

tredition was established in 2006 by Sandra Latusseck and Soenke Schulz. Based in Hamburg, Germany, tredition offers publishing solutions to authors and publishing houses, combined with worldwide distribution of printed and digital book content. tredition is uniquely positioned to enable authors and publishing houses to create books on their own terms and without conventional manufacturing risks.

For more information please visit: www.tredition.com

TREDITION CLASSICS

This book is part of the TREDITION CLASSICS series. The creators of this series are united by passion for literature and driven by the intention of making all public domain books available in printed format again - worldwide. Most TREDITION CLASSICS titles have been out of print and off the bookstore shelves for decades. At tredition we believe that a great book never goes out of style and that its value is eternal. Several mostly non-profit literature projects provide content to tredition. To support their good work, tredition donates a portion of the proceeds from each sold copy. As a reader of a TREDITION CLASSICS book, you support our mission to save many of the amazing works of world literature from oblivion. See all available books at www.tredition.com.

 Project Gutenberg

The content for this book has been graciously provided by Project Gutenberg. Project Gutenberg is a non-profit organization founded by Michael Hart in 1971 at the University of Illinois. The mission of Project Gutenberg is simple: To encourage the creation and distribution of eBooks. Project Gutenberg is the first and largest collection of public domain eBooks.

Benign Stupors A Study of a New Manic-Depressive Reaction Type

August Hoch

Imprint

This book is part of TREDITION CLASSICS

Author: August Hoch
Cover design: Buchgut, Berlin – Germany

Publisher: tredition GmbH, Hamburg - Germany
ISBN: 978-3-8472-2249-1

www.tredition.com
www.tredition.de

Copyright:
The content of this book is sourced from the public domain.

The intention of the TREDITION CLASSICS series is to make world literature in the public domain available in printed format. Literary enthusiasts and organizations, such as Project Gutenberg, worldwide have scanned and digitally edited the original texts. tredition has subsequently formatted and redesigned the content into a modern reading layout. Therefore, we cannot guarantee the exact reproduction of the original format of a particular historic edition. Please also note that no modifications have been made to the spelling, therefore it may differ from the orthography used today.

BENIGN STUPORS

THE MACMILLAN COMPANY

NEW YORK · BOSTON · CHICAGO · DALLAS
ATLANTA · SAN FRANCISCO

MACMILLAN & CO., Limited

LONDON · BOMBAY · CALCUTTA
MELBOURNE

THE MACMILLAN CO. OF CANADA, Ltd.

TORONTO

BENIGN STUPORS

A STUDY OF A NEW MANIC-DEPRESSIVE REACTION TYPE

BY
AUGUST HOCH, M.D.
LATE DIRECTOR OF THE PSYCHIATRIC INSTITUTE OF THE
NEW YORK STATE HOSPITALS, WARD'S ISLAND, NEW YORK.
LATE PROFESSOR OF PSYCHIATRY, CORNELL UNIVERSITY
MEDICAL COLLEGE, NEW YORK
New York
THE MACMILLAN COMPANY
1921

All rights reserved

PRINTED IN THE UNITED STATES OF AMERICA

Copyright, 1921,
By THE MACMILLAN COMPANY
Set up and printed. Published July, 1921.
Press of
J. J. Little & Ives Company
New York, U. S. A.
TO
MY FORMER COLLEAGUES
IN THE
NEW YORK STATE HOSPITAL SERVICE

EDITOR'S PREFACE

A word should be said as to the origin and history of this book. When the late Dr. Hoch became Director of the Psychiatric Institute of the New York State Hospitals in 1910, he found there an interest in just the kind of psychiatric research which it was his ambition to further. His predecessor, Adolf Meyer, had developed the conception that the psychoses should be looked on as psychobiological reactions rather than rigid nosological entities and had inculcated the habit of scrupulously thorough examination and record of what the patient said and did. Meyer had broken away from the sterile habit of making diagnoses in accordance with the set terms used to label symptoms; and his work and that of his assistants thus led to a collection of valuable material which could serve as a useful starting point for the keen clinical investigation of Hoch. Specifically, attention had already been fixed on the study of the so-called functional psychoses, comprising what are generally termed Dementia Præcox and Manic-Depressive Insanity. An urgent problem in this field was to separate different reaction types in order to discover which were recoverable and which chronic or progressive. In order to understand psychological reactions, interrelation rather than [viii] mere coincidence of symptoms must be studied and, to aid in this, free use was made of the fundamental principles of unconscious mentation as exposed in the theories of Freud and his followers.

Almost at the outset it had been discovered that many patients presented clinical pictures that would not fit into existing diagnostic pigeon holes. Dr. George H. Kirby, whose skill and industry had made the most valuable contributions to the archives of the Institute, published in 1913 a brief paper in which he pointed out, not only that many cases with "catatonic" symptoms recovered, but also that clinically the behavior of stupor showed it to be related to manic-depressive insanity as well as dementia præcox. Dr. Hoch took up the problem at this point. Using Dr. Kirby's material and adding to it his earlier observations as well as current cases, he endeavored to work out the essentials of the stupor reaction. It was his ambition to describe stupor not only in its psychiatric bearing but also as a life reaction.

The significance of this task is to be realized only when one considers the general import of the functional psychoses. They are, biologically, failures of adaptation. The chronic and deteriorating cases give up the struggle permanently, while the temporary insanities lay bare the soul of man as he catches a glimpse of unreality but turns back to face the world as it is. When one realizes that emotional disturbances are characteristic of the benign psychoses, it is easy to imagine how much such studies [ix] may ultimately illuminate the problems of normal life.

The technical value of this work to psychiatry is more immediate. Kraepelin laid the foundations for systematic classification with his dementia præcox and manic-depressive groups. But the rigidity of the latter, allegedly descriptive, term has confused the problem of classifying many benign psychoses. It was Hoch's ambition to prove that, although elation and depression were the commonest mood anomalies in this group, they had no more theoretic importance than anxiety, distressed perplexity or apathy. These other moods, although less frequent, are just as characteristic of the psychoses in this group. In other words, the name "Anxiety-Apathy Insanity" would be as appropriate, theoretically, as Kraepelin's term. In 1919 Hoch and Kirby published a report on the perplexity cases. This present book was designed to show that the symptom complex centering around apathy is as distinct as that which is recognized by all psychiatrists as mania with its predominant characteristic of elation.

In 1917 ill health forced Dr. Hoch to resign from his official duties. He retired to California with the purpose of adding to psychiatric literature the fruits of his long experience and unrivaled judgment. His first task was this book. In the midst of this work came a sudden collapse. As I had been in close touch with his researches, coöperating in psychological speculations, and was free to devote [x] some time to it, he asked shortly before his death that I complete the book. This obligation is incommensurate with the debt I owe for years of inspiration, tuition and criticism.

The task has been mainly literary. I found the first five chapters practically completed, while it has not been difficult, as a rule, to discover from his copious notes what his intentions were as to the details of the following chapters. I have been greatly aided by the assistance of Dr. Adolf Meyer and of Dr. Kirby. The latter has been good enough to read the entire manuscript, making invaluable suggestions and criticisms.

John T. MacCurdy.

New York.

TABLE OF CONTENTS

CHAPTER

    Editor's Preface
- I. Introduction and Typical Cases of Deep Stupor
- II. The Partial Stupor Reactions
- III. Suicidal Cases
- IV. The Interferences with the Intellectual Processes
- V. The Ideational Content of the Stupor
- VI. Affect
- VII. Inactivity, Negativism and Catalepsy
- VIII. Special Cases: Relationship of Stupor to Other Reactions
- IX. The Physical Manifestations of Stupor
- X. Psychological Explanation of the Stupor Reaction
- XI. Malignant Stupors
- XII. Diagnosis of Stupor
- XIII. Treatment of Stupor
- XIV. Summary of the Stupor Reaction
- XV. The Literature of Stupor

    Index

BENIGN STUPORS

CHAPTER I
INTRODUCTION AND TYPICAL CASES OF DEEP STUPOR

The fact that psychiatry lags in development and recognition behind other branches of medicine is due in part to the crudity of its clinical methods. The evolution of interest in science is from simple, obvious and tangible problems to more intricate and impalpable researches. Refined laboratory work has been done in psychiatric clinics, particularly along histopathological lines, but clinical studies follow antiquated methods. The internist does not say, "The patient has sugar in his urine, therefore he has diabetes and therefore he will die." He finds a glycosuria and looks for its cause. If this symptom is found to be related to others in such a way as to justify the diagnosis of diabetes, a therapeutic problem arises, that of adjusting the chemistry of the body. The prognosis depends not on the disease but the interreaction of the organism and the morbid process. Both in diagnosis and treatment an individual factor, the patient's metabolism, is of prime importance. Now in psychiatry, although the personality is diseased, this personal factor has been [2] almost entirely neglected. Text-books furnish us with composite pictures which are called diseases, not with descriptions of reactions brought about by the interplay of personal and environmental factors. Educated people are not satisfied with novels that fail to depict real characters. Clinical psychiatry, however, has been content with the dime-novel type of character delineation. This is all the more disappointing, inasmuch as the study of insanity should contribute largely to our knowledge of everyday life. This defect can only be remedied by looking on every case as a problem in which the origin of each symptom is to be studied and its relation traced to all other symptoms and to the personality as a whole. This is an ambitious task and we do not pretend to any great achievement, merely to a beginning.

No better psychoses could be chosen for a preliminary effort than benign stupors. Every psychiatrist has seen them, although they are wrongly diagnosed as a rule, and they play no small rôle in the world's history. Euripides represents Orestes as having a stupor which is pictured as accurately as any modern psychiatrist could describe an actual case. [1] St. Paul is chronicled as falling to the ground, being thereafter blind and going without food or drink for three days. While apparently unconscious he had a religious vision. St. Catherine of Siena had several unquestionable stupors, which are fairly well [3] described. In fact the mystics in general seem to have had communion with God and the saints most often when they seemed unconscious to bystanders. [2] The obsession with death, which seems so intimate a part of the stupor reaction, is a fundamental theme in poetry, religion and philosophy. The psychology of this interest is, speaking broadly, the psychology of stupor. So, from a general standpoint, our problem is related to the study of one of the most potent ideas which move the soul of man.

Psychiatrically, stupors have long remained an unsolved riddle. In the century prior to 1872 (See the digest of Dagonet's publication in Chapter XV) French psychiatrists wrote some good descriptions of stupor and offered brilliant, though sketchy generalizations about the condition. Two years later an English psychiatrist (Newington, See Chapter XV) improved on the French work. Little light has been thrown on the subject since then. The researches of the later French School showed that stupor often occurs in the course of major hysteria, but this left many of these episodes obviously not hysterical. When serious attempts were made at classification, this ubiquitous symptom complex was hard to handle. Wernicke wisely refrained from attempting more than a loose descriptive grouping. He called all conditions with marked inactivity and [4] apathy "akinetic psychoses" and said that some recovered, some did not. Taxonomic zeal began to blind vision when Kahlbaum formulated his "Catatonia" and included stupor in the symptom complex. The condition which we call stupor occurs in the course of many different types of mental disease. It is true that it is frequent in catatonia but is not exclusively there. Mongols have black hair and straight hair, but one cannot therefore say that any black and straight haired man is a Mongol. Fortunately Kahlbaum prevented serious error by leaving the prognosis of his catatonia open. When Kraepelin included it in his large group of Dementia præcox, however, it implied that stupor could not be an acute, recoverable condition. [3] He unquestionably advanced psychiatry greatly but his scheme was too ambitious to be accurate. Many observers saw patients, classified as dements according to Kraepelin's formulæ, return, apparently normal, to normal life. Finally Kirby [4] published a series of cases which showed decisively that this classification was too rigid.

Since his paper is the foundation for this present study, it should be reviewed carefully. He first points out that Kraepelin's "Dementia præcox" [5] includes much more than it should with its inevitably bad prognosis. He shows how others have found patients with catatonic symptom complexes proceed to recovery and speaks of these symptoms occurring in epilepsy and even in frankly organic conditions, such as brain tumor, general paralysis, trauma and infections. Kirby's first claim is that there are probably fundamentally different catatonic processes, deteriorating and non-deteriorating. Lack of knowledge has prevented us from understanding the meaning of the symptoms and hence making the discrimination. He points out that stupor seems to represent an attitude of defense, similar to feigned death in animals, and that in a number of his cases it was clear that the stupor symbolized the death of the patient. Apparent negativism, he found to be often a consciously assumed attitude of aversion towards an unpleasant emotional situation. In cases where there had been no prodromal symptoms pointing definitely to dementia præcox the outcome was almost always good. To discriminate the cases with good outlook from those with bad, he discerned no difference in the stupors themselves, but observed that the mental make-up and initial symptoms differed sufficiently for diagnosis to be made. His most important point is, perhaps, that these benign stupors showed a definite relationship to manic-depressive insanity in that some patients passed directly from stupor to typical manic excitement, while in others a "catatonic" attack replaced a depression in a circular psychosis.

[6] Kirby introduces, then, the idea of stupor being a type of reaction which can occur either in dementia præcox or in manic-depressive insanity. The matter cannot be left there, in fact it raises

new problems: what constitutes the reaction? how are the various symptoms interrelated? are they different in deteriorating and acute cases? what is the teleological significance of the reaction? if it be an integral part of the manic-depressive group, how does it affect our conceptions of what manic-depressive insanity is? More than five years have been spent in endeavors to answer these questions and the results of the study are now presented.

Naturally the first point to be settled is: what constitutes the stupor reaction itself. We can say at the outset that it is seen in the purest form in benign cases, hence they make up the material of this book. To discover the symptoms of the disorder one cannot do better than to study them in their most glaring form in deep stupors, where consistently recurring phenomena may be assumed to be essential to the reaction.

Case 1.—*Anna G.* Age: 15. Admitted to the Psychiatric Institute July 25, 1907.

F. H. The mother and two brothers were living and said to be normal. The father died of apoplexy when the patient was seven.

P. H. The patient was sickly up to the age of seven, but stronger after that. It is stated that she got on well at school, though she was somewhat slow in her work. She was inclined to be rather quiet, even when a child, a bit shy, but she had friends and was well liked by others. After recovery she made [7] a frank, natural impression. She was always rather sensitive about her red hair. She began to work a year before admission and had two positions. The last one she did not like very well, because, she alleged, the girls were "too tough."

Three weeks before admission she came home from work and said a girl in the shop had made remarks about her red hair. She wanted to change her position, but she kept on working until six days before admission. At that time her mother kept her at home as she seemed so quiet, and when the mother took her out for a walk she wanted to return, because "everybody was looking" at her. For the next two days she cried at times, and repeatedly said, "Oh, I wish I were dead—nobody likes me—I wish I were dead and with my father" (dead). She also called to various members of the family, saying she wanted to tell them something, but when they came she would only stare blankly. For a day she followed her mother around, clung to her, said once she wanted to say something to her, but only stared and said nothing.

Four days before admission she became quite immobile, lay in bed, did not speak, eat or drink. She also had some fever.

The patient herself, when well, described the onset of her psychosis as follows: She knew of no cause except that her brother, some time before the onset (not clear how long), was run over by an automobile and had his foot hurt. She claimed that while still working she lost her ambition, lost her appetite, did not feel like talking to any one; that when she went out with her mother it merely seemed to her that people stared at her. The day before she went to the Observation Pavilion her cousin came to see her, and she thought she saw, standing beside this cousin, the latter's dead mother. She also thought there was a fire, and that her sister was sweeping little babies out of the room. Then, she claimed, she felt afraid (this still on the day before going to the Observation Pavilion) because she had repeated visions of an old woman, a witch. This woman said, "I am your mother, and I gave you to this woman (i.e., patient's real mother) when you were a baby." She also was afraid her mother was "going away."

At the *Observation Pavilion* she was described as constrained, staring fixedly into space, mute, requiring to be dressed and fed.

[8] *Under Observation:* 1. For five months the patient presented a marked stupor. She was for the most part very inactive, totally mute, staring vacantly, often not even blinking, so that for a time the conjunctivæ were dry. She did not swallow, but held her saliva; did not react to pin pricks or feinting motions before her eyes. Sometimes she retained her urine, again wet and soiled the bed. Often there was marked catalepsy, and the retention of very awkward positions. As a rule she was quite stiff, offering passive resistance towards any interference. She had to be tube-fed at first. Later she was spoon-fed, and then would swallow, in spite of the fact that during the interval between her feeding she would let saliva collect in her mouth. For a time she had a tendency to hold one leg out of bed, and when it was put back would stick the other out.

Sometimes she walked of her own accord to the toilet chair, but on one occasion wet the floor before she got there.

During the first month after admission, this stupor was interrupted for two short periods by a little freer action: she walked to a chair, sat down, smiled a little, fanned herself very naturally when a fan was given to her, though even then did not speak.

There was, as a rule, no emotional reaction, but after some months she several times wept when her mother came, though without speaking. Once when taken to the tub she yelled.

Her *physical condition* during this stupor was as follows: She menstruated freely on admission, then not again until she was well. Several times she had rises of temperature to 102° or 103° with a high pulse and respiration; again a respiration of 40, with but slight rise of temperature, though the pulse had a tendency to go to 130 and over. She was apt to show marked skin hyperæmia wherever touched. With the fever there was found a leucocytosis of from 11,900 to 15,000, with marked increase of polynuclear leucocytes (89%). She got very emaciated, so that four months after admission she weighed 68 lbs. (height 5' 2").

2. About five months after admission she was often seen smiling, and again weeping, and she began to talk a little to the nurses, though not to the doctors. She also began to eat excessively of her own accord, and rapidly gained weight, so that [9] by January she weighed 98½ lbs., a gain of 30 lbs. in two months. Yet she continued to be sluggish.

3. For two more months she was apathetic and appeared disinterested, often would not reply, again, at the same interview, she would do so promptly and with natural voice. This condition may be illustrated by the summary of a note made on January 29, 1908, which is representative of that period. It is stated that she sat about apathetically all day, appeared sluggish, but was fairly neat about her appearance and cleanly in her habits. There was at no time any evidence of affect, except when asked by the examiner to put out her tongue so that he could stick a pin in it she blushed and hid her face. When asked whether she worried about anything, she denied this. When questions were asked, she sometimes answered promptly and in normal voice, again simply remained silent in spite of

repeated urging. On the whole, it seemed that simple impersonal questions were answered promptly; whereas difficult impersonal questions or questions which referred to her condition were not answered at all. She proved to be oriented. Thus she gave the day of the week, month, year, the name of the hospital, names of the doctors and nurses promptly. She also counted quickly and did a few simple multiplications quickly. But she was silent when asked where the hospital was located, how long she had been here, whether she was here one or six months, how she felt. Questions in regard to the condition she had passed through, or involving difficult calculations, she did not answer. However, some questions regarding her condition asked in such a way that they could be answered by "yes" or "no" were again answered quite promptly. Thus when asked whether her head felt all right she said, "Yes, sir." (Is your memory good?) "Yes." (Have you been sick?) "No, sir." (Are you worried?) "No."

4. This apathy cleared up too, so that by the middle of March she was bright, active and smiled freely. With the nurses she was rather talkative and pleased, though this was not marked. Towards the physician only was she natural and free. She then gave the *retrospective account* of the onset detailed above. When questioned about her condition she claimed not to remember the Observation Pavilion, although recalling vaguely going there in a carriage. She was almost completely amnesic for a consider [10] able part of her stay in the Institute. She claimed it was only in November or December that she began to know where she was (five months after admission). In harmony with this is the fact that she did not recall the tube- and spoon-feeding which had to be resorted to for about four months of this period. No ideas or visions were remembered. As to her mutism she said, "I don't think I could speak," "I made no effort," again "I did not care to speak." She claimed that she remembered being pricked with a pin but that she did not feel it. She remembered yelling when taken to the tub (towards end of the marked stupor) and claimed she thought she was to be drowned.

When she went home (March 24, 1908) she got into a more elated condition. She was talkative, conversed with strangers on the street, said to her mother that she was now sixteen years old and wanted "a fellow." When the mother would not allow her to go out, she said it would be better if they both would jump out of the window and kill themselves. She then was sent back to the hospital. In the first part of this period after her return, she was somewhat elated and overtalkative, though she did not present a flight of ideas, and was well behaved. She soon got well, however, and was discharged, four months after her readmission, fully recovered.

After that, it is claimed, she was perfectly well and worked successfully most of the time with the exception of a short period in the spring of 1909, when she was slightly elated.

In 1910 she had a subsequent attack, during which she was treated at another hospital. From the description this again seems to have been a typical stupor (immobility, mutism, tendency to catalepsy, rigidity). According to the account of the onset sent by that hospital (it was obtained from the mother), this attack began some months before admission, with complaints of being out of sorts, not being able to concentrate and fearing that another attack would come on. Finally the stupor was said to have been immediately preceded by a seizure in which the whole body jerked. She made again an excellent recovery.

The patient was seen about two years after this attack, and described the development of the psychosis as follows: She claimed she began to feel "queer," "nervous," "depressed," got sleepless. Then (this was given spontaneously) she suddenly [11] thought she was dying and that her father's picture was talking to her and calling her. "Then I lost my speech." As after the first attack, she claimed not to have any recollection of what went on during a considerable part of the stupor but recalled that she began to talk after her brother visited her. It is not clear how she was during the period immediately following the stupor.

She made a very natural impression and came willingly to the hospital in response to a letter and was quite open about giving information.

Case 2.—*Caroline DeS.* Age: 21. Admitted to the Psychiatric Institute June 10, 1909.

F. H. The father died of apoplexy when patient was nine. The mother had diabetes. A paternal uncle was queer, visionary.

P. H. The patient was always considered natural, bright, had many friends, and was efficient.

Some months before admission the patient's favorite brother, who is a Catholic, became engaged to a Protestant girl, and spoke of changing his religion. The family and the patient were annoyed at this, and the patient is said to have worried about it, but was otherwise quite natural until seven days before admission. Then, at the engagement dinner of the brother, the psychosis broke out. She refused to sit down to the table, and then suddenly began to sing and dance, cry and laugh and talk in a disconnected manner. Among other things, she said "I hate her," "I love you, papa" (father is dead), "Don't kill me." She struck her brother. She was in a few days taken to the Observation Pavilion.

The patient stated after recovery that what worried her was that the brother would marry a Protestant and that he would leave home (favorite brother).

At the *Observation Pavilion* she was excited, shouted, screamed, laughed, called out "Don't kill me," again "Brother, brother," "You are my brother" (to doctor).

Under Observation: 1. On admission, and for two weeks, the patient presented a marked excitement, during most of which she was treated in the continuous bath. She tossed about, threw the sheets off, beat her breasts and abdomen, put her fingers into her mouth, bit the back of her hands, waved her arms about, [12] sometimes with peculiar gyration, etc., at the same time shouting, singing, again praying, laughing or crying, sometimes fighting the nurses and resisting them. She also talked quite a little as a rule, but there were periods when, although excited, she would not talk or answer questions. She was very little influenced in her talk by the environment. When on one occasion asked if she had any trouble, she said: "No—I don't want, somebody else gave me a book—all right I love myself, Uncle Mike too—all right too—all right I am in Bellevue—I love everybody except the Jews all right, all right—give me water, give me milk, give me seltzer—white horse uncle—Holy Father, he is killing me, I want my mother," or "Wait a minute, say, that's a lie—oh no, Holy water—no I didn't wash the water away—oh, she forgets, I am sick—mother why don't you come—look at the baby, they knocked my head against the wall—wait a minute, isn't that terrible?—I was married—I was so—I forgot—April fool—I kiss you seven kisses and one more—I love papa and mamma, I like others too—I am papa's angel child—yes I confess I love him, but I don't want to die myself." On another occasion, when asked where she was, she said: "I am at the ball—I am going to Heaven—don't shoot me" (affectless). (Why are you afraid?) "Because you see—high water (in the tub)—white horse." (What about the water?) "My name is Caroline—if you love me, father, tickle me under my feet," or, rolling her eyes up, "Oh, isn't that awful, that ring, that diamond, that is the key to Heaven."

2. For about ten days she was somewhat different. She became quieter and at first lay muttering unintelligibly, saying some things about being killed, but speaking little, often restlessly tossing about and tremulous. She had to be tube-fed. On one day (July 1) she smiled more and talked more, said to the physician "You have been arrested for me—you arrested the first man that I ever—New York State—let me see that book" (note pad). Then she went on: "Oh, I am all apart—diamonds—they didn't know—must I keep them clean?—what is your name?—that is another thing I would like to know." But when asked what house she was in she said: "This is the same Ward's Island" and then added, "How long have I been here?—there is my picture up there (register), who is that? (listening) it's Ida [13] ..." She began to sing softly. Then again she whined. "O mamma, mamma!" When asked how long she had been here, she said: "Since Decoration Day, when my father went in my sister's house, nobody could catch up with me—somebody blackened her eyes." When asked whether she was sick, she said "No, insane."

Although, as was stated, she said at one time, "This is the same Ward's Island," usually questions regarding orientation were not answered, as she gave few relevant replies, but she repeatedly said spontaneously that she was in "Hoboken or Bellevue," and called the nurse by the name of a former teacher. A few days after this state had developed she had a fever. Once this rose to 104°. The fever lasted two weeks, coming down gradually. It was associated with a leucocytosis of 15,000 on June 29 (no differential count) and with coated tongue. No Widal (two examinations). No diazo (July 1).

3. Then while the temperature still lasted she developed a stupor which persisted for about a year. During this time her temperature rose to 100° without ascertainable cause. She lay for the most part motionless, changing her position but rarely; her expression was stolid; she retained and drooled saliva, wet and soiled herself. She never answered any questions; showed no interest whatever. At times she was quite stiff and very resistive but never cataleptic. Her extremities were cold and cyanotic. She had to be tube-fed throughout. During this time she lost much hair.

After some months she occasionally gazed about furtively, or later watched everything when unaware of being observed; at this time she also smiled occasionally at amusing things, or perhaps said "yes" or "no" to questions, but usually was stolid when interrogated.

Then about nine months after admission, while in the condition just described, she developed a lobar pneumonia. During it she remained the same. But during convalescence she began to speak and eat.

4. A period followed lasting six months during which she was up and about, but sat or stood around a good deal. On the other hand, she helped the nurses a little when urged. Her face was often stolid, again she looked about. At times (even [14] nearly to the end) she drooled and soiled. She said little. At no time was she resistive. On other occasions she smiled or laughed, not always on provocation, or she showed little playful tendencies, such as throwing a pillow about the room, tearing leaves from the plants, taking the doctor's arm and walking down the hall, asking him to kiss her. At such times she often looked quite bright, keen, alert and amused. Towards the end she would give at times playful answers, such as "I came to-day," or "This is the Hall of Fame." This tapered off, so that by December, 1910, she was perfectly well.

Retrospectively, the patient claimed not to remember the upset at the dinner, or what happened afterward, although recalling the trip to the Observation Pavilion. She denied any memory of the journey to the hospital, but could tell what ward she came to. How well the condition after that was recalled, was not inquired into, except that she could or would not explain further the utterances during the first period. For the stupor period it is stated that she remembered many external facts, but it is not clear in which period they occurred.

Catamnestic Note. May, 1913: She has worked efficiently, and is said to have been perfectly well.

Case 3.—*Mary F.* Age: 21. Admitted to the Psychiatric Institute June 28, 1902.

F. H. The mother died when the patient was five. The father was living, an alcoholic and reckless man. Four brothers and sisters died in infancy.

P. H. The patient was the only surviving child. She was brought up in a convent and orphan asylum until 11, when her father remarried. At 12 she had to go to work, hence she had but little education. She was bright, efficient, well liked by her employers (in one position five years). As to her peculiarities, she was thought to be, perhaps, a little headstrong, and was also described as always very exact, rather quick-tempered and inclined to be irritable when crossed.

She was married six months before admission and had a *baby three weeks before admission*. The husband stated that when the father found out she was pregnant, he spoke of killing him. He frequently upbraided both husband and wife, though he lived [15] with them. Even after the child was born he continued to be disagreeable.

The patient was rather low spirited and quieter after her marriage. She worried over her illegitimate pregnancy and the scolding from her father. But nothing was thought of all this, and it did not interfere with her activity. The birth was normal. She had no flow, no unfavorable symptoms, and sat up on the twelfth day. She is said to have appeared natural mentally.

A week before admission the family returned from the christening, having left the patient apparently well. They now found her sitting in her chair, limp, with closed eyes, giving no answer to questions. Only after about twenty minutes could she be aroused. After her father had given her milk with whiskey in it, she claimed he had poisoned her. In the evening she was bright and lively, singing and dancing with the others, but in the night she woke up her husband, seemed frightened, said somebody was in the room and that he should get a priest as she was going to die. The husband went to sleep again. The next forenoon the patient claimed she had been frightened all night and thought her father was going to kill her husband.

On the second day, while sitting at breakfast, she groped about for the bread plate for some time and then said she had been blind for a short time. During the day she had frequent spells in which she would close her eyes, become perfectly quiet and difficult to rouse. Sometimes at the beginning of these spells she would say "I am going." She was then taken to her aunt and walked there, a distance of a few blocks. She was there for two days before going to the Observation Pavilion. In this time she is said to have been quiet for the most part, often apparently sleeping or staring. Once she said she was "rather dirty, filthy." Once she tried to get out of the window, said it was a door and that she wanted to get out and take a walk. Above all, she had, in these two days, repeated peculiar seizures which the aunt and the husband described as follows: When sitting on a chair she would close her eyes, clench her fists, pound the side of the chair, get stiff, slide on the floor, then thrash her arms and legs about and move the head to and fro. She frothed at the mouth. After the attack, which lasted a few minutes, she breathed heavily for a while. Once she wiped off the froth [16] with a handkerchief and gave the latter to the aunt, saying "Burn that, it is poison." Before the attack she sometimes said that it got dark over her eyes and that her face felt funny, again that she had a pain in the stomach which worked towards her right shoulder. There was no cry in the beginning of the attack, but once she wet herself.

After recovery the patient herself told the development of her psychosis thus:

There was trouble between the father and the husband, and she was afraid of her father. On the day of the christening she took sick: a queer feeling came over her and she wondered whether she was going to die, "Then I seemed to lose myself, and when I came to I found my family standing around me." Her father gave her whiskey and she thought it was poison. "That night I had spells of dancing and singing, it must have been something I took, perhaps the liquor." The same night she was frightened, thought her father might do some harm, and had a vision of a person in white standing at her bed. After that she had repeated spells in which she knew nothing until "I came to again." "It was a queer trembling."

At the *Observation Pavilion* she was described as in a state of "intense mental depression," taking no interest in things going on about her. She spoke, however; said she wanted to die, that she had imagined her father had given her poison, that every one was against her, and that people were talking about her.

1. *On admission* the patient had a slightly elevated temperature, which soon subsided, full breasts but without inflammation. Sordes were not mentioned.

For a few days she was essentially somewhat restless, getting out of bed, disarranging her clothes, wandering about—all in a rather deliberate, aimless way, sometimes vaguely resistive, again with free movements. She looked, dazed, sometimes stared straight ahead and looked "dreamy." Occasionally there was a tendency to close her eyes. With the restlessness she looked at times "a little apprehensive," or shrank away when approached. She spoke slowly, with initial difficulty, but answered quite a number of questions. The mental content of this period was displayed in the following utterances: She would ask for a priest, or say "Have I done something?" or "Do people want [17] something?" or, when asked why she was here, she said "I have done damage to the city, didn't I?" (What have you done?) "I don't know." Or she spoke of people watching her. When asked the day, she said "Judgment Day," yet she knew the month. Once when asked what the place was she said, "This is the hereafter." When asked what had happened at home, she said: "Voices told me I was to be killed." She was not clearly oriented, called the place Bellevue, asked "Isn't this a hospital?" yet again said, "Ward's Island, where they work." On the day of admission she thought she came "the day before," but knew she had come in a boat. When asked her address, she said slowly, "Didn't I live at, etc.," giving the address correctly. To the physician she said, "Are you my brother?" And on another occasion, "My God! You are Charlie" (brother). It was difficult to get her to eat, and she had to be spoon-fed.

2. Then she became more preoccupied, the restlessness was much less in evidence, it became necessary to tube-feed her, she retained her urine, answered a few questions, and when asked where she was, she said, "Calvary, ain't it?" (What house?) "Heaven, ain't it?" She still called the physician by the name of her brother. After a few days this gave way to a more marked stupor which lasted nearly two years. This was characterized most frequently by a complete inactivity. She usually lay or sat motionless, sometimes with mouth partly open, letting the flies crawl over her face, gazing in one direction, soiling, wetting, resisting moderately or markedly any interference, and had to be tube-fed. But this was not the invariable state. The most constant feature was her mutism, but even that was a few times interrupted. Thus, when after a visit from her uncle (towards the end of July, 1902) she tried to get out of the window and was prevented, she swore at the nurse. Or in August, 1902, when she got into another patient's bed and was taken out, she resisted and said promptly: "I think it is a damned shame I can't get into my own bed." But this was the extent of her talk for a year and a half. Nor was she always totally inactive. In the middle of July, 1902, she sometimes tried to get out of bed, wandered about, got into other patients' beds. It was on such an occasion that the above incident happened. In August, 1902, she sometimes tried to get out when the door was opened, and [18] we have seen that she tried to get out of the window, but she did not change her placid expression at such times. Her motive was not known. On two occasions towards the end of 1902, when she was taken to a dance and was made to take part, she waltzed with considerable animation but did not speak. This was quite striking in that these incidents occurred in a setting of marked inactivity (i.e., a condition in which she had to be pushed to the table, pushed to the closet). She did not soil any more, but she sometimes drooled and had to be spoon-fed. However, on a third occasion when this was tried, she had to be dragged around. Finally, though her facial expression showed at times a preoccupied staring, she more often looked around, sometimes quite freely and often looked up promptly enough when accosted. But there was very little evidence of any affect at any time. We have seen that twice she swore a little when opposed. On another occasion she slapped a patient when the latter helped her. Twice she was seen crying a little without apparent provocation, but she did not laugh,

and the only suggestion of pleasurable emotion was that at the two dances mentioned she could be led into a certain animation. Usually, even when she got less resistive towards the end, she was essentially apathetic.

Once in January, 1903, she could be made to write her name but wrote her maiden name. In the end of 1903 she improved gradually (a condition not well observed), so that by December she answered some questions in a low tone. Even in April, 1904, she was still described as apathetic, though she had begun to do some work.

3. Then she improved markedly and began to work, looked after herself in a natural way, spoke freely, was entirely oriented and her mood generally presented nothing striking. But her mental attitude was still peculiar when she was questioned. She seemed somewhat inattentive, sulky, sneering. Thus, when asked why she was here, she said, "You will have to ask those who brought me here."

She denied ever having been pregnant, said the nurses on the ward had spoken of her having had a child and that they had showed her a child (one was born on that ward about August, 1903) but that it was not hers. She thought it was wrong for the nurses to speak on the ward of her having been pregnant. [19] Again questioned about her marriage, she first said she had not been married, again that she was married "a year ago" (was in the hospital then). Again she spoke of her husband as her "gentleman friend," claimed she called herself Mary M. (maiden name) until a girl friend wrote her a letter addressed to Mrs. F. From then on, she called herself by her married name. But she thought that probably they sometimes spoke of her marriage in fun. If she were Mrs. F. she would be living in Mr. F.'s house.

On June 29, when again asked about her marriage, she said she was to have been married in December (correct date). (Were you?) "So they say." (Do you remember it?) "In a way." (When was the baby born?) "You will have to ask somebody more superior to me, more experienced." Then, when further questioned about the age of the baby, she said, "The baby I saw in the ward was about a year old," and she claimed not to remember ever having a baby. When asked why she had come here she said, "Well, I don't know, perhaps you know better, through sickness I guess," and later: "Well, don't you ever get a cold and want doctors to examine you?" (What kind of a place?) "This is a nice place for sensible people who have enough knowledge to know and realize what they come for." But she knew the name of the place, the date, the names of persons.

Questioned about the trouble with her father or her husband's trouble with him, she denied it, "If he did (sc. have any trouble), I don't remember." About her not speaking, she said, in answer to questions, "I didn't know what I was here for, what was the object in keeping me here"; and to other questions about her condition, "I don't know, those who examined me can tell you more about that." Finally, she said in reply to the question, why she came here, "I don't remember *unless it was through fire*," but would not explain what she meant.

In the beginning of July, she again said that she had no recollection of her marriage.

She then improved a great deal and finally appeared very natural, gave the retrospective account noted in the history, had a clear appreciation of the fact that she was married and had a child. She claimed that she had previously forgotten about her marriage and thought she was still merely keeping company with Mr. F. She claimed not to remember coming to the hospital, [20] did not know what ward she came to, who the doctor and nurses were, in fact claimed that it was about a year before she knew where she was. But she remembered having been tube-fed. She could not say why she did not speak. But she appreciated that she had been ill.

Ten years after discharge the husband, in answer to an inquiry, stated that she had been perfectly well and had had no trouble at three successive childbirths.

Case 4.—*Mary D.* Age: 20. Admitted to the Psychiatric Institute September 17, 1907.

F. H. The grandfather and the father of the patient were alcoholics. The father died three years before the patient's admission; he was killed in an accident. The mother stated that she herself was nervous, but she made a normal impression.

P. H. The patient was described as bright at school and efficient in her work as a dressmaker, but she was rather quiet, inclined to stay at home and had not much inclination to consort with the other sex. She was rather proud. As an example of this is stated the fact that she was always somewhat sensitive, because the family lived in the basement of the house in which her mother was janitress. She did not menstruate until 16. It was about this time that her father was killed in an accident. She was considerably upset by this, talked a good deal about the way he was killed, but did not break down. The patient on recovery stated that it worried her because the father died without having any chance to get a priest.

Six weeks before admission the patient was given a vacation, as there was not work enough in the shop, but she worked at home.

Two or three weeks before admission her appetite failed somewhat, and ten days before admission, without any appreciable cause, she began to sleep badly, seemed somewhat nervous, became a little "fidgety" and said she worried because her mother had to work so hard. Later she began to speak about people saying that the ambulance would come for her and she heard voices saying "You will be dead." It is not known in what emotional setting these remarks were made. Her mother took her to a dispensary. On the way she asked the mother where she was going and said [21] "I can't tell the number and I don't know where I am going. I think I am losing my mind." She also said she could not understand any more what she read. She was put to bed. She then talked less, appeared stupid, and was inclined to refuse food.

Four days before admission she claimed that she could see her dead father beckoning to her, again she said a certain young man was God. She was sent to the Observation Pavilion. On the day she went there she was reported to have shown a slight jaundice.

The patient, after her recovery, added to the above account of the mother, that about two weeks before admission, for no reason which she could state, she began to feel quiet, and that after that her father's death began to prey on her mind, and that later she had a vision of her father. She claimed that in this period she had no fear but that her head felt dizzy and her vision seemed dim.

At the *Observation Pavilion* the patient was described as constrained, refusing food, mute, resistive of attention, sometimes muttering to herself and having the appearance of uneasiness.

Under Observation: 1. On admission the patient had a slight jaundice, which disappeared in a few days, and the bile test in the urine was negative on admission. She was rather thin, but otherwise in good physical condition. Her temperature was 99.2°.

For three months the patient was very inactive, moving very little. She had to be dressed and undressed, when taken out of bed. She often was markedly constrained, either lying with her head raised from the pillow, or for long periods of time holding her arms or hands in rather constrained positions on her body. But there was at no time any catalepsy when tested by moving her arms. In the beginning, however, before she lay so persistently with her head raised, she was found holding it up from the pillow after her hair had been fixed. Again, she did not correct other, rather uncomfortable, positions in which she had been left. There was also at times a slight or occasionally a somewhat more marked resistance in her arms and neck, but this never amounted to a pronounced resistance. She sometimes did not react to pin pricks, sometimes flinched a little, never warded off the pin, indeed she would put out her tongue repeatedly when asked to do so in order to have a pin stuck into it. She very [22] often wet and soiled, once even immediately after she had been taken to the closet, on which occasion she did not urinate. Her face was usually dull, vacant and immobile, but sometimes, when questioned or when something obtrusive happened, a little puzzled. Occasionally she looked slowly about or followed people with her eyes. There was no evidence of any affect as a rule, but not infrequently she smiled, even quite freely at times, when the physician came to her or on other appropriate occasions. For example, once when a nurse came into the ward whom she had known outside she flushed and smiled a little. Once when the mother came to see her a few tears appeared, the only time this occurred.

Although for the most part immobile, when she did move, she was distinctly slow. When asked to do certain things, she usually did not comply, but now and then, after urging, would show her tongue after delay, or merely open her mouth; or she would bring the hand forward slowly when the physician offered his hand in greeting. Once she fumbled with her braids slowly. When out of bed, she stood about aimlessly or sometimes walked somewhat slowly.

She was almost entirely mute, but a few times she returned a greeting quite promptly, or on another occasion (September 23) she said quite promptly, when asked how she felt, "I feel better. I took off my clothes" (correct—she had been up and put to bed again). Again she sometimes answered simple questions by "yes" or "no," though sometimes in a contradictory and rather aimless manner, but promptly enough. Once she said to her mother, "I can't, I have to remain here." There were some other replies which we shall presently take up. Several times it was possible to make her write. On these occasions she wrote her name promptly, or might write only after much delay or stopping in the middle of a word.

This leads us to her capacity to think, the defect of which was perhaps most clear in her writing. Thus, though having been told to write her name, and having written it quickly enough, when, immediately after it, she was asked to write her address or the name of the hospital, she had to be urged much, and then wrote each time merely a repetition of her name, this time much more slowly. On October 13, when she was asked to write her [23] name, she wrote it correctly; then for the address she wrote the house number correctly, but for 90th street she wrote "90theath"; and, urged again for the address, she added "Dr. Wyeth." Again when asked to write the word "watch" she was slow, and finally put down "10." When on October 23 she was asked to write "Manhattan State Hospital," she wrote "Manhatt Hhospshosh," and for "Ward's Island" (which she was told), "Ww Iland." Then she was asked to write "I wish to go home." She wrote "I wish to go home, go West." Here again the first part was written promptly.

We now can add some of the other replies which she gave. Once she was asked "Do you know where you are?" She promptly said, "Yes." (Where?) No reply. On another occasion, at the initial examination, she said she was home or "in papa's house." Once when asked "Do you know me?" she said "Yes." (What is my name?) "Miss D." (her name). On the occasion on which she had stated that she had taken off her clothes, she was asked "Where have you taken off your clothes?" She made the irrelevant reply, "That was the girl the one I had."

2. Then she improved somewhat. On January 5 she walked about a little more, though slowly, and still looked slightly puzzled when questioned. She spoke more readily, counted promptly though once stopped in the middle of the exercise. In calculation she multiplied correctly 3 × 7, but for 4 × 9 repeated the 21, and when given 9 × 9 she did not answer. A few days later, though she lay again motionless with her head raised as before, and, as she had sometimes done, smiled brightly when accosted, she gave few replies, but when asked to write down the month she slowly wrote "December." Asked to write it the second time, she did it promptly. She also replied promptly by saying "Yes" when asked whether Christmas, and again whether New Year's, had passed, but did not reply to the questions how long ago Christmas, or how long ago New Year's, had occurred. On January 23 she was decidedly more free and prompt in her replies, yet she still wet and soiled (in fact this did not cease until the end of the month, when great improvement occurred). At this time she gave quite a number of calculations promptly, about an equal number wrongly. She knew where she was, knew the names of a number of people about her, but thought she had [24] been here about two weeks (four months), and gave the year and the date, the latter as the 28th of January. When then told that it was Thursday, January 23, and that she must remember it, and asked five minutes later what she had been told, she again said "January 28" and left out Thursday. To some questions to which she did not know the answers, since she had an amnesia for the time of their occurrence (the incidents of coming here), she simply remained silent. Even on February 7, when she was much freer, helped the nurses, and said herself she was "smarter," she had difficulty in thinking, said she was 17 (21), gave the date of her birth correctly, but the current year as 1909 (1908) and still insisted she was 17. She then did the calculations on paper, and with considerable difficulty got correctly "22." But she could not straighten out the discrepancy. At that time, also, she still wrote "Hospitital," calculated even simple multiplications with some mistakes, could not get the point of a story, and to retention tests gave poor results. Indeed, even seven days later, when she wrote a very rational letter and appeared quite natural, she made some omissions in her writing, and a few mistakes in spelling.

However, she now improved rapidly, and by March 31 she made a very natural impression, was frank, free, had good insight, calculated well, etc., understood a story, retention was good.

She then gave the retrospective account embodied in the history, and in addition told that she had no recollection of going to the Observation Pavilion, the coming here, or the first part of her stay, including presentation of the case at a staff meeting, a physical examination and a blood examination, and she claimed for a long time not to know where she was, "I was in a kind of dazed condition." She also said she could not understand the questions which were asked her. This probably refers, however, to the second part, i.e., the partial stupor lasting for two months. She did not "feel like talking," the limbs "felt stiff-like."

Case 5. — *Annie K.* Age: 22. Admitted to the Psychiatric Institute January 7, 1907.

F. H. The father was an alcoholic, who died when patient was a child. A paternal aunt had a nervous breakdown, with recovery. The mother appeared to be normal.

P. H. The mother stated that the patient was a rather delicate child. She attended school irregularly, never felt much interest in it, and was always glad to be at home and help the mother take care of the other children. On the other hand, she is said to have been quite lively, rather a tomboy, with a temper. She left school at 14; learned dressmaking for a year, but did not get along well. Then she took several other positions, which she held for about a year, getting on pretty well.

She married at 20. Her husband never supported her well and often beat her. She had to borrow money to get along and worried much. During pregnancy she seemed to worry more, had crying spells, and often seemed absorbed in thought.

Three weeks before admission she gave birth to a child. The labor was somewhat difficult, but she had no fever. She got up on the tenth day, and then seemed to lose all interest, did not attend to the baby, said she was not strong enough. She sat about, appearing depressed. The mother then took her and the baby to her house. There she sat or walked about, said very little. But she repeatedly came to her mother, said she had something to tell her, or that she had "done something," although she could never be induced to say what. Once she came to her and said, "You are not going to die." She often moaned. Finally, she claimed a neighbor had been saying she was poisoning the baby.

The patient herself gave, after recovery, the onset as follows: When she married she knew her husband was not what he should be, but not that he was so bad as he proved to be. He was a gambler, did not support her, and this caused her much worry. When she became pregnant, eight months after marriage, this increased her worry, and throughout the pregnancy she spoke much to a neighbor about her worries, and said she did not know how she could manage, pay the doctor, and the like, but she did not say much about it to her mother (because the latter would have made such a fuss about it, or would have said, "It serves you right"). Then the childbirth came. This further accentuated her worries. She felt her difficult circumstances, wondered how she could get the necessary money, "I lay there worrying." And she claimed she did not sleep at all. About her statement, mentioned by the mother, that she had done something, she said that [26] she thought she had poisoned the child by giving it fennel tea, and that she thought a neighbor who visited her said she had poisoned it. She was then put to bed again, and one night she had a vision of her father. This frightened her. She thought this meant he had come for her and she wanted to die.

At the *Observation Pavilion* she was dull, staring, resisting attempts at passive motions.

Under Observation: 1. There was nothing noteworthy in her physical condition, except for a rise of temperature to 100° occasionally during the first month of her admission. For the first four months she was often found lying in bed with her head half raised from the pillow, or standing or sitting about in constrained positions, immobile, frequently she let saliva collect in her mouth. She usually wet and sometimes soiled the bed. Sometimes, when sitting in a constrained position, she let herself gradually slide on the floor. She often began to feed herself when urged, but would not finish, and had to be spoon-fed, as a rule. She was never tube-fed. She was often quite stiff and showed marked resistance. This was manifested either when passive motions were tried, at which times she usually resisted passively, i.e., she became more tense; or when there broke through a more active aggression and she would strike. Above all, the opposition showed itself towards the nurses' attention; in this she also showed either a passive, aimless opposition and stiffness, or a more active one; but even in the latter an open show of angry affect, or plain irritation, though present at times, was by no means constant. When it was present, she would strike quite aimfully; once she struck the nurse and said, "You are the cause of it all," and once, when the nurse tried to give her some milk, she said, in an irritated tone, "I wonder people would not let me alone some time." Again, she bit a patient who tried to hold her. On another occasion she quickly jumped up and pulled the hair of a patient who evidently disturbed her by her noisy shouting. As was stated, she usually wet the bed, resisted being taken to the toilet, or when taken there, would not urinate or defecate, but would do so as soon as she was returned to bed; or she urinated while standing. The same perverse opposition was seen when she would refuse a glass of milk, but grab it when [27] it was taken away and then refuse to let go. She often would grasp the bedclothes or other things and hold on aimlessly.

She rarely spoke, answered almost no questions, complied, as a rule, not even with the simplest commands. To pin pricks she did not react except at times by flushing. But she did not stare, rather looked about, and was at times easily attracted by noises or happenings about her, and would then look in that direction not without some interest. Often there was then an expression of bewilderment. Her mood, however, was, as a rule, apathetic, but at times, as stated, she showed some anger. Once she wept, and a few times she smiled or snickered. As a rule, this happened without appreciable cause. But once, when a cheering remark was made, she smiled; or, when her picture was taken (to show the peculiar constrained attitude with the head raised from the pillow), she laughed loudly.

Although she spoke rarely, she made a few utterances in the first few days. Thus she suddenly said: "I want to see Mr. N.—what I said to him was not right," or "Listen! there are the priests calling," or "You are all faking—it is me that done it—they are all dressing up downstairs," or "I told you she was not able to nurse the baby," or "I have nobody, I am lost—I want to know the truth—my mamma," or she called her sister, "They are dead since last night."

Even during the more stuporous state she could, a few times, be made to write a little. Then she either wrote very slowly and not more than a letter, or if she wrote more, it was remarkably mixed up. Thus when asked to write the date, she wrote, "Jane (mother's name) to me to Chrichst," or when asked to write her name: "Annie take you ktusto."

As to her orientation, nothing could be made out as a rule. At first, however, a few weeks after admission, she spoke correctly of the month as January and spoke of the Island. When at that time she was asked if she had a baby, she said, in an annoyed tone, "I don't know."

2. In the beginning of May, i.e., four months after entrance, her condition changed somewhat, and for two months she presented the following state: She stood about, or walked around slowly, usually with her arms folded. She had a tendency to stand near the door. She had to be assisted in dressing, pushed [28] rather than led to her meals, and urged to eat. For the most part, she would not answer questions, but would either smile in a sneering way, or just walk away, or say, "Oh, don't bother me," or "I don't want to talk," and generally her attitude was rather sulky. Nor was this only towards the physicians but towards the husband, sister and child as well. When on May 17 the sister came, she would not speak to her but said "Go away." The baby she simply pushed away sulkily when it was brought to her. To the husband she said on May 31, "Go away, you stink." In the first part of this period, she presented some bursts of elation, on one occasion turned somersaults, indulged in a few pranks with laughter, or once, when a knock at the door was heard, she called out "Holy gee, cheese it, the cop." But these occurred only in the first part of the period. On June 1 she spoke to the nurse, said, "What is the matter with these people, they must be crazy," asked to go home, and was then by the nurse found to be oriented, and to know the names of people around her. But when she was asked about the baby she would not answer, and questioned whether she was not married, she said "I don't know."

Yet when the physician desired to talk to her, she was just the same as before and remained so for two more weeks. Another somewhat isolated occurrence was when on June 18 she spoke a little to the physician, but she sat in a constrained position when taken into the office and answered many questions by "I don't know," namely, those regarding her condition and feelings, the questions about orientation, about her mother's address, and her child's age; but when asked how long she had been married she said correctly "Two years."

At the beginning of July she improved quite rapidly, and on July 5 appeared fairly free and gave a fair retrospective account, with some urging, and it was thought that she smiled somewhat too freely. However, on July 27, she seemed perfectly well, had normal insight, and then gave the second retrospective account, which, together with the first, will now be taken up.

Retrospectively: She claimed to remember things at home, and at both interviews said she recalled being taken to the Observation Pavilion. While there she thought she knew where she was, remembered that she did not talk. She had a feeling she [29] was going to die and said "I thought I would die if I kept still." However, the transfer to this hospital was vague in her mind, as was the entrance on the ward, and she claimed not to have known for quite a while where she was. She added that she used to wonder where she was, how she had gotten here, and how she could get out, and thought the questions which were asked were queer. Individual occurrences, too, specifically inquired into were not recollected, such as an examination in a special room. Of the mixed-up writing at the end of the second week, she had no recollection even when it was shown to her. She did not recall having her picture taken (with eyes open) two months after entrance. Yet a sudden angry outburst ten weeks after admission was remembered. She stated that she struck the patient because the latter annoyed her by her shouting. She had a general recollection of being stiff, having her head raised, and of soiling and drooling, but could not account for it. She felt stubborn. She also claimed not to have been hungry and not to have felt pin pricks.

In regard to ideas which she had, she claimed to be afraid at first that she would be cut up. She remembered repeated visions of her father at night, also once of her dead aunt, who said "Come to me." She thought she was in a cemetery, all the family were dead, the baby dead. In the beginning, too, she sometimes heard a priest whom she had known, say "Be good and God will look after you."

In regard to the later period, she recalled that she got up in May and felt cross. She did not answer because she did not want to be bothered. She pushed the baby away because she did not think it belonged to her, the husband because she did not like him. (She did not think she was not married.) She evidently remembered the visits, thought she knew where she was, knew she stood near the door "because I wanted to go home." Besides the idea that the baby was not hers, she recalled none, and thought she had no hallucinations.

She was discharged perfectly well six months after admission to the hospital. Soon after that, she left the husband, once had him arrested in 1908 and sent to the workhouse. She was again examined in 1913, and was found to be perfectly well, and she stated she had been well since the discharge.

[30] These five cases will have to suffice for the present. They were given in full in spite of the fact that we shall leave out of our present considerations the history of the cases and certain of the stages, and confine ourselves to that stage of each case which is best qualified to give us a good general survey of the essential features of the stupor reaction.

These phases are: stage 1 of Case 1, lasting five months; stage 3 of Case 2, lasting one year; stage 2 of Case 3, lasting two years; stage 1 of Case 4, lasting three months; stage 1 of Case 5, lasting four months.

We gather from these descriptions that the essentials of the stupor reaction are (1) more or less marked interference with activity, often to the point of complete cessation of spontaneous and reactive motions and speech; (2) interference with the intellectual processes; (3) affectlessness; (4) negativism.

Inactivity: There is a complete cessation or more or less marked diminution of all spontaneous or reactive movements. This includes such voluntary muscle reflexes as contain a psychic component. For instance, there is, often, an interference with swallowing (letting saliva collect and drooling), winking, and even with the inhibitory processes used in holding urine and feces (soiling and wetting). Often there is no reaction to pin pricks or feinting motions. The inactivity also often interferes with the taking of food so that spoon-feeding or tube-feeding has to be resorted to. The patient may keep his eyes cov [31] ered or stare vacantly, the face often presenting a remarkably immobile wooden, or stolid, expression. Complete mutism is the rule. When activity is not totally interfered with, those movements which are present may be slow. The patient may have to be pushed around and be able to take a few steps, but soon relapses. More often they are of normal rapidity. Speech then may also be slow and low, but usually shows no change except for the fact that it is diminished in amount. Sometimes awkward positions are assumed and retained, and there may be catalepsy.

Negativism: A common symptom is perverse resistiveness. It may consist in a marked stiffening of the body which is assumed spontaneously or appears only when attempts at interference are made, or there may be a more active turning away or even a direct warding off, sometimes with scowling or anger or even swearing and striking. Retention of urine, which is seen at times, should, perhaps, be mentioned here. Now and then we find that a patient is put on the toilet and cannot be induced to urinate or defecate, while soiling and wetting occur at once on returning to bed.

The intellectual processes: Little is known about the intellectual processes from direct observation in these more pronounced cases, except for the fact that in Case 5 questions or obtrusive occurrences sometimes produced a somewhat puzzled facial expression. Moreover, the patient retrospectively stated that she was unable to understand the ques [32] tions, which points to marked difficulty in apprehension. We also find that occasionally there is evidence of an interference with the intellectual processes which showed itself in what may be called "paragraphic" writing when the patient could be induced to write. Above all, we see that retrospectively very little is remembered of what took place during the stupor, even of such obtrusive events as the moving from one ward to another, tube-feeding, physical examination, the presentation at a staff meeting, and the like.

Affect: Complete affectlessness is an integral part of the stupor reaction. Modification of the statement will later be mentioned. The patient is indifferent so far as his basic condition is concerned, and it is only by certain stimuli that at times emotional reactions can be elicited, some tears at a visit of a relative, an appropriate smile at a joke or a comical situation when the stupor is not too deep or an angry reaction called forth by interference.

Catalepsy: Waxy flexibility or merely a tendency to maintain artificial positions is a frequent but not an essential symptom.

Physical Condition: Not infrequently we find in the beginning or in the course of the stupor an elevation of temperature to 101°, 102° or even 103°. In one case we found a marked cyanosis in the extremities. Case 2 showed marked loss of hair. Gain in weight is never observed and marked emaciation is the rule. This we may attribute to the refusal of food.

[33] A perusal of these cases, then, shows that the dominant (and well-nigh exclusive) symptoms of the stupor are inactivity, apathy, negativism and disturbance of the intellectual functions. Benign stupor can be defined as a recoverable psychosis characterized by these four symptoms. The meaning of such vague physical manifestations as the low fever is not clear.

Footnotes:

[1] MacCurdy has discussed the psychological phenomenon of a dramatist depicting a psychosis correctly in "Concerning Hamlet and Orestes." *Journal of Abnormal Psychology*, Vol. XIII, No. 5.

[2] Many of these states seem to be hysterical rather than manic-depressive stupors, but so far as the unconsciousness goes, there is probably as much psychological as symptomatic resemblance between the two types of reaction.

[3] Kraepelin recognizes, of course, the occurrence of stupor symptoms or states in the course of manic-depressive psychoses. It is stupor as a clinical entity, as a separate psychosis, that he regards

as one form of the catatonic, and therefore of the dementia præcox, reaction.

[4] Kirby, George H.: "The Catatonic Syndrome and Its Relation to Manic-Depressive Insanity." *Jour. of Nervous and Mental Disease*, Vol. 40, No. 11, 1913.

CHAPTER II
THE PARTIAL STUPOR REACTIONS

The cases thus far considered, namely, those of marked stupor, are fairly well known and have been studied by others. Less well known and formulated, but even more important from a practical as well as from a theoretical point of view, are what may be called partial stupors.

The reader has noted that the states of deep stupor described in the last chapter, did not end abruptly with a sudden return to health or a sudden change to another type of psychosis. They all gradually passed away, not by the disappearance of one symptom after another, but by the attenuation of all. Sometimes a more or less stable condition persisted for months, in which there was no stupor in a literal, clinical sense but when apathy, inactivity, interference with the intellectual functions and negativism all existed. Had these been the only states observed in these patients, there might have been some ground for doubt as to the diagnosis. As it was, it was clear that we were dealing with mild stages of stupor. When a psychiatrist meets with an undeveloped manic state, he calls it a hypomania and does not hesitate to make this diagnosis in the [35] absence of complete development into a florid excitement. This procedure is not questioned, because the manic *reaction* as distinguished from a *mania* is well recognized. We believe that there is just as distinctive a *stupor reaction* which may be exhibited either in deep stupors or what we may term partial stupors. Theoretically, complete apathy, inactivity, etc., make up the clinical picture of a deep stupor. When these symptoms appear rather as tendencies than as perfect states, a partial stupor is the product. That partial stupors occur as well-defined psychoses, developing and disappearing without the appearance of deep stupor, we shall attempt to show in the following three typical cases:

Case 6.—*Rose Sch.* Age: 30. Admitted to the Psychiatric Institute August 22, 1907.

F. H. Both parents were living (father 74, mother 68), as were two brothers and two sisters. All were said to be normal.

P. H. Nothing was known of the patient's early characteristics, except that she herself said she was slow at learning in school and did not have much of an education. But when well she made by no means the impression of a weak-minded person. The husband had known her for ten years. He married her eight years before admission, by civil process, keeping this from his own family because he was a Jew and she a Christian. He said that this undoubtedly worried the patient at times and that she often asked him when he would take her to his family. The patient herself later also said that this used to worry her. Finally, one and a half years before admission she agreed, on account of the children, to accept the Hebrew faith, and they were then married in the synagogue. But he still did not take her to his family.

There were four pregnancies: the first child died; of the survivors one was 8, a second 5 years old. Finally, a year before [36] admission, she became again pregnant. During the pregnancy one of the children had whooping cough and she herself was thought to have caught it. The baby was born three months before admission. It was a blue baby which died two days after birth. The patient flowed heavily for three weeks and was taken to a hospital, where she continued to flow intermittently for some weeks more.

Finally, three weeks before admission, a hysterectomy was performed. Several days after this, when the sister-in-law visited her, the patient begged her to take her home, said the doctor wished to shoot her and to give her poison. Later the patient confirmed this, saying that she thought they wanted to give her saltpeter, and that she heard them say they wanted to shoot her.

When taken home she refused food; gazed about, was absorbed, seemed obstinate, and several times tried to jump out of the window. Retrospectively the patient stated that she heard children on the street call "Katie." She thought they meant her child, heard that it was to be taken away from her, and a similar idea again came out later in her psychosis, namely, that somebody was going to harm her children.

At the *Observation Pavilion* she appeared stupid, rather immobile, her attention difficult to attract.

Under Observation: On admission the patient appeared sober, impassive, moved very little, was markedly cataleptic, though not resistive. On the other hand, her eyes were wide open and she looked about freely, following the movements of those around her not unnaturally. When questioned, she looked at the questioner rather intently, and was apt to breathe a little more rapidly, and made some ineffectual lip motions but no reply. To simple commands she made slow and inadequate responses. She flinched when pricked with a pin, but made no attempt at protecting herself. She had to be spoon-fed. The catalepsy persisted only for two days.

After this she continued to show a marked reduction of activity, moved very little, said nothing spontaneously, had at first to be spoon-fed (later ate naturally enough). But she never soiled herself and went to the closet of her own accord.

Emotionally she seemed dormant for the most part, though for the first few days she appeared somewhat puzzled, and one night [37] when a patient screamed she seemed afraid and did not sleep, whereas other nights she slept well. She answered only after repeated questions and in a low tone. Very often, though her attention was attracted easily enough, her answers were remarkably shallow and also showed a striking off-hand profession of incapacity or lack of knowledge. This was often without any admission of depression or concern about her incapacity. She would usually say "What?" or "Hm?" or repeat the question, but most often would say, "I don't know," this even to very simple questions. For instance, when asked, "What is your name?" she answered, "My name? I don't know myself" (but she did give her husband's name), or when asked to write her name, she said, "I don't know how to write," or "Call Annie, she will write my name." When requested to read or write (even when asked for single letters), she would make such statements as "I can't read." However, she finally named some objects in pictures. This condition was characteristic of her for two weeks.

Then her condition changed a little. She spoke a little more freely but was similarly vague. The following interview of September 9, is characteristic: When asked how she was, she said, "Belle." (Are you sick?) "No." (Is your head all right?) "Yes." (Is your memory all right?) "Yes." (Do you know everything?) "Yes." (Understand everything?) "Yes." (Are you mixed up?) "No." (Do you feel sick?) "No." But when asked where she was, how long she had been here, what the name of the place was, what was the occupation of those about her, she said, "I don't know." (How did you come here?) "I couldn't tell how I came up here." (What are you here for?) "I am walking around and sitting on benches," but finally, when again asked what she was here for, she said, "To get cured." She now gave and wrote her name and address correctly when requested, also gave the names of her children. Yet when asked about the age of the girl, said, "I don't know, my head is upside down." When an attempt was made to make her repeat the name of the hospital, or the date, or the name of the examiner, she did so all right, but even if this was done repeatedly and she was asked a few minutes later, she would say "I couldn't say," or "I forget things," or "I have a short memory," or she would give it very [38] imperfectly, as "Manhattan Island," or "Rhode Island" for "Manhattan State Hospital, Ward's Island." (How is your memory?) "All right." But when at this point the difficulty was pointed out, she cried. (Why?) "Because I forget so easily." All this was while her general activity was much reduced, and she seemed to take very little interest in her surroundings.

Then she improved somewhat, asked the husband some questions about home, and on one occasion cried much and clung to him and did not want to let him go without taking her. She also began to work quite well, but still said very little spontaneously. During this period when asked questions, she spoke freely enough, but seemed somewhat embarrassed. What was still quite marked were striking discrepancies in giving dates, and her utter inability to straighten them out when attention was called to them, as well as to her inability to supply such simple data as the ages of her children. Her capacity was later not gone into fully but it was certainly less defective on recovery than at this time. She was rather shallow in giving a retrospective account during this period. Even later, when she had developed a clear insight and made, in respect to her activity and behavior, a natural impression, she was not able to give much information about her psychosis, although she apparently tried to do so.

She was discharged recovered four months after admission, her weight having risen from 93 lbs. on admission to 133 lbs. on discharge. For the first two weeks of her stay in the hospital, her temperature varied between 99° and 100°.

Retrospectively: She said in answer to questions about her inactivity and difficulty in answering that she did not feel like talking, felt mixed up, could not remember well, did not want to write.

Before she was quite well she knew of her entrance to the Observation Pavilion and her transfer to Ward's Island, of which she could give some details, but thought she had been in the Observation Pavilion two weeks instead of three days and in the admission ward one month instead of a few hours. As to the precipitating cause of the attack, she spoke of her flowing so much after childbirth and of her operation.

[39] She was seen again in March, 1913, when she seemed quite normal mentally and claimed that she had been well ever since leaving the hospital.

With the exception of negativism, which appears only in the anamnesis, all the cardinal stupor symptoms are found in this history. Particularly noteworthy is her intellectual deficiency which seemed to be made up of a real incapacity plus a remarkable disinclination for any mental effort whatever. It is important to note that her attitude towards this disability was usually one of indifference and that, in general, there was no show of affect whatever. Freedom of speech was the last thing for her to regain.

Case 7.—*Mary C.* Age 26. Single. Admitted to the Psychiatric Institute April 7, 1907.

F. H. The father had repeated attacks of insanity, from which he recovered, but he died in an attack at the age of 60. A sister also had a psychosis, from which she recovered.

P. H. The patient was rather quiet and easily worried. When 14 she had some dizzy spells, with momentary loss of consciousness. After that time she had no such attacks, except after a tooth extraction when about 24.

The patient came to the United States six months before admission. She went to live with a cousin who died a week after she arrived at his house. She worried and said that she brought bad luck. Then she took a position, where she was well liked, but she was not particularly efficient. In this situation she often felt homesick and lonely.

Two weeks before admission an uncle died, which affected her considerably. She spoke of his leaving three children, and would not go to the funeral. Then she thought she was going to die. She felt dizzy, weak, walked with a stooped position, was sleepless. In the midst of this she suddenly felt frightened and walked [40] into her mistress' room, to whom she complained that some one was talking outside but could not tell what was said. She heard shooting. Retrospectively, after recovery the patient said that at that time she suddenly got "mixed up," and that her "memory got bad."

She was taken to a general hospital, where she thought there was a fire, and screamed "Fire!" She was soon transferred to the *Observation Pavilion*, where she appeared dazed, moving slowly, yet showing a certain restlessness. She spoke of "the boat" being shut up so that no one could go out. Again, she said "The boat went down and all the people keep turning up." Retrospectively the patient stated about this condition that she remembered going to the general hospital but not her stay at the Observation Pavilion. (The trip to the Manhattan State Hospital was again clearer to her.) About the ideas she had at the time, she remembered only that the room seemed to go around, and that after she had come to the Manhattan State Hospital and was clearer, she thought she was in Belfast, was on a ship, and that people were drowning.

Under Observation: On admission she had a temperature of 100°, a coated tongue, suffused conjunctivæ. There were herpes of the lower lip, a general appearance of weariness and exhaustion, a flushed face, trace of albumen in the urine, which was absent on the third day, no leucocytosis, but 41 per cent. lymphocytes.

Then and henceforth she was inactive and very slow in all her movements; she never stirred spontaneously, and had to be pushed to the toilet and to the table; she ate slowly. She did not speak spontaneously, and her replies were very slow in coming. She had to be urged considerably before she would speak and, as a rule, she did not answer. On one occasion she was for a day totally inactive and looked duller. That day and on a few other occasions she wet the bed. There was at times an appearance of dull bewilderment. When, soon after admission, asked whether she felt cheerful or downhearted, she said "downhearted," but this was the only time. Often she answered "I don't know," when asked whether she was worried, and she could never say what she was worried about. Again she directly denied worry. Sometimes she smiled appropriately, and repeatedly, [41] when asked how she felt, said, "I feel better." In answer to questions as to how her head was, she replied several times, "My memory is gone," also "I can't take in my surroundings," or "I don't know where I am," or "I cannot realize where I am." Again, she spoke of being dizzy and once said it was as though the room went round. Sometimes she knew where she was or knew names, again said "I forget," but she always was approximately oriented as to time. There were no special ideas expressed and no hallucinations, except in the very beginning when she still thought at night, when she heard the boats on the East River, that people were being drowned. She later, as stated above, said she thought she was on a boat and people were being drowned.

By June, i.e., two months after admission, she began rhythmical swaying of the body, twisting of the fingers, or pulling out some of her hair. She ascribed this behavior simply to "nervousness."

On July 16, after a visit from her cousin, who said to her that if she worked she would soon get better, she began spontaneously to occupy herself somewhat. She became more active, said she felt stronger and brighter, and that her memory was better. By the beginning of August she was fairly free, but still spoke in a rather low voice, although answering well. Her capacity to calculate also remained poor. When asked about the more inactive state, she said she had been afraid to stir. (What afraid of?) "I didn't know where to go or what to do." Further, she recalled that she had had a numb feeling in her tongue, could not speak quickly, and that her mind had felt confused and "she could not take in things." Further review with her of the earlier period of her psychosis showed that there was a blank for external events and most of the internal events during this time.

She made a perfect recovery and was discharged August 7, 1907, four months after admission.

This case, although very like the last, differs from it in two particulars. For one day her symptoms were sufficiently marked to suggest a deep stupor. Secondly, her intellectual incapacity was not so marked (always approximately oriented for time) [42] and with this there was some subjective appreciation of her defect. Apparently, however, this insight did not cause her any worry. The affectlessness was equally prominent in both of the foregoing cases, the fact that Mary C. (Case 7) once admitted feeling downhearted in response to leading questions, having little significance in the face of her expression, actions and usual denial of worry. It is interesting to note that, during the bulk of her psychosis, her only complaints were of mental hebetude and dizziness. Possibly the latter was merely an expression of her subjective confusion.

Case 8.—*Henrietta H.* Age: 22. Admitted to the Psychiatric Institute March 6, 1903.

F. H. The father stated that both parents were living and well, also eight brothers and sisters.

P. H. The patient came to this country when she was a baby. She was bright at school and industrious. From the age of 17 on, she worked in a drygoods store and gave satisfaction. About her mental make-up no data were available, except for the statement that she always made a natural impression.

When 21 (February, 1902), without known cause, she broke down and was sent to the Manhattan State Hospital, but was not observed in the Institute ward. She remained in the hospital for three months. It was claimed that the attack came on suddenly two days before she was sent away. She suddenly appeared anxious, said something had happened and became excited. This lasted for about a week, and then she was, as the description says, "depressed and cataleptic." She remained in this condition for about a month, during which time there was a slight rise of temperature. Then she improved gradually and was discharged three months after admission. After recovery from the present attack the patient stated that during the first sickness she had visions of dead friends.

She was perfectly well in the interval.

[43] Six days before admission she suddenly became excited, refused to eat, and began to talk, repeating phrases over and over. Then she became elated and excited.

After recovery the patient described the onset of her psychosis as follows: Six days before admission, after having been perfectly well and without any known cause, she was feverish and vomited, but slept well. Next day she felt nervous, and her thoughts were clear. She constantly thought of dead friends, heard them talking, when she tried to do anything the voices said, "Don't do that." She also thought somebody wanted to harm her people. Soon she started singing and felt happy.

Then she was sent to the *Observation Pavilion*, where she appeared to be in the same condition which was observed in the Institute.

Under Observation: 1. On admission she was in good physical condition, except for her skin seeming greasy. She presented for nine days the following picture: She was essentially elated, laughing, singing, jumping out of bed, good-natured and tractable, and very talkative. Her productions showed a good deal of sameness and a certain lack of progression. She spoke at times in a rather monotonous voice, but again often in very theatrical tones, with much, rather slow, gesturing. The following are very representative samples:

"I have been suffering from my own blood, my own blood sent all away from home. I just came from Bellevue. I left here last May (correct) a healthy girl. A sister is a sister—I wonder why shorthand is shorthand, a stenographer is a stenographer (seeing stenographer write)—a kind brother, Bill H.—why H. his wife is a sister-in-law to us, she has four children—four beautiful children—sister-in-laws and brother-in-laws—telephone ringing (telephone did ring)—dear Lord, such a remembrance—remembrance was remembrance, truth was truth—honesty is honesty—policy is policy—if she married him, she is my sister-in-law and he is my brother-in-law—Max knows me—she changed her name to Mrs. R.—two children who are Rosie and Maud, if names were given, names should not be mistaken—they are Julia, Lillian—Rosie and Maud—why should wonders wonder and wonders cease to wonder, why should blunders blunder and blunders still blunder; sleep is one dream and dream means sleep [44] —if move is moving, why not move?" When she accidentally heard the word wine, she said "Guilty wine is not in our house—wine is red and women are women, and women and wine and wine and women and wine and song." Again, "You are not Mr. Kratzberger, Mr. Steinberger, Mr. Einberger—you are not Mr. Horrid or Mr. Storrid—perhaps you are Mr. Johnson or Mr. Thompson—no, you are Dr. C." (correct).

She was quite clear about her environment.

Although the mood was throughout one of elation, on the ninth day in the forenoon she cried at times, wanted to see her mother, and spoke in a depressed strain (content not known). A few hours after that she suddenly became quiet.

2. Then for four days (March 14-17) she was markedly inactive, though at times got out of bed. She looked about in a bewildered manner, did not speak spontaneously, but could with urging be induced to make some replies. She did this now fairly promptly, now quite slowly. Questions were apt to bring on the bewilderment. Thus, when asked where she was, she merely looked more bewildered, finally said "Bellevue—I don't know," and questioned who the doctor was whom she had called by name in her manic state, she said, with some bewilderment, "Your face looks familiar." (Where have you seen me?) "In New York." She claimed to feel all right. There was no real affect. She made the statement that at home she heard voices saying "You will be killed."

3. Henceforth this bewilderment ceased, and for 16 or 17 days she was essentially inactive for the most part, for a short time with a tendency to catalepsy and some resistiveness, and at that time lying with eyes partly closed. As a rule she said nothing spontaneously, but replied to some questions, usually with marked retardation, again more promptly. She constantly denied feeling sad or worried, repeatedly said she felt "better," only on one occasion did she cry a little. When asked to calculate she sometimes did it very slowly, again fairly promptly. The simple calculations were usually done without error, the others with some mistakes. As to her orientation the few answers obtained showed that at times she knew the name of the place and the day, again she gave wrong answers (Bellevue).

Once asked on March 23 for the day, she said April. She wrote her name promptly on one occasion, again a sentence slowly but without mistakes. Once during the period she sang at night. Once she suddenly ran down the hall but quickly lapsed into the dull condition.

On April 4, at the end of this period, she suddenly laughed, again ran down the hall, said she had done nothing to be kept on Ward's Island. But she quickly lapsed again into the dull state. Later, on the same day, when the doctor was near, she said, in a natural tone, "Thank God, the truth is coming out." (What do you mean?) "That I have been trusting in a false name and that Miss S. (the nurse) should not nurse me." Then she got suddenly duller, calculated slowly and with some mistakes, 3×17=41, 4×19=56, and when asked to write Manhattan State Hospital she wrote (not very slowly) "Mannahaton Hotspalne."

4. Next day it was noted that she was more stuporous, and she remained so for two weeks, now showing a decided tendency to catalepsy and more resistance than before, though not marked, except in the jaw. She lay often with head raised, sometimes with eyes partly open, or staring in a dull, dreamy way, neither soiling nor drooling, however; a few times she looked up when spoken to sharply. There was no spontaneous speech. Usually she did not answer at all, but a few times a short low response was obtained. Once she wrote slowly a simple addition, put down on paper. When, on one occasion, asked how she felt, she, as before, said, "I feel better."

5. Then, with the exception of a day at the end of the month, when the more stuporous state was again in evidence, she returned to her former condition without catalepsy or resistiveness and without staring, but essentially with inactivity or slowness. She now even dressed herself, answered slowly though not consistently, but she again denied feeling troubled or sad, "I feel better."

On July 7 she got brighter but was still rather slow. She then even began to do some work. She again denied feeling sad.

In a few weeks, while having a temperature of 102° with vomiting and diarrhea, she suddenly got freer. She then said, in answer to questions, that she did not speak because she was not sure whether it would be right, again because she seemed to lose her speech. She did not move because she was tired, had a [46] numb feeling. She said she had not been sad, "but I had different thoughts," "saw shadows on the walls of animals, living people and dead people." She was not frightened, "I just looked at them." People moved so quickly that she thought everything was moved by electricity. She thought her head had been all right.

After a few days she relapsed into a duller state again, but then got quite free and natural in her behavior. On August 28 she gave a *retrospective* account of her psychosis, a part of which has been embodied in the history. She had insight in so far as she knew she had been mentally ill. She claimed to remember the Observation Pavilion and her coming to the hospital, also the incidents during the manic state, when she heard cannon and thought a war was on, and voices she could not recognize nor understand. Then she became stupid, although neither sad nor happy.

Then, she claimed, she got stupid, but neither sad nor happy. She claimed to have known all along where she was, but felt mixed up at times, her thoughts wandered and she felt confused about the people. She thought she was in everybody's way, thought others wanted to get ahead of her, did not speak because she did not know if it were right or wrong, felt she might cause disturbance if she answered. (It is not clear whether she had complete insight into the morbid nature of these statements.) She also claimed again that all along she "saw shadows on the wall," "scenes from Heaven and Earth," "shadows of dead friends laid out for burial." She had insight into the hallucinatory nature of these visions. Sometimes she thought she was dead also. She claimed that she began to feel better when these shadows stopped appearing in June (the actual time of her improvement).

She was discharged recovered a month later, after having been sent to another ward.

In this case, then, we find that the two months of stupor were ushered in by a brief state in which, in addition to the usual inactivity, there was a certain bewilderment, increased by questions, while the [47] orientation which in the preceding manic state had been good became seriously interfered with. The psychosis bordered on deep stupor for brief periods when the inactivity seemed to be complete or she lay in bed with her head raised from the pillow. On the other hand, there were occasional sudden spells of free activity even with a certain elation. She could often be persuaded to answer questions or to write, the slowness of this spoken or written speech varying considerably. Her replies revealed the fact that she was essentially affectless and that her intellectual processes were interfered with, even to the extent of paragraphic writing. We have, therefore, here again features similar to those of the preceding cases. In addition we must add as important that this patient said retrospectively that she thought she was dead, that she saw "shadows from Heaven and Earth," "shadows of dead friends laid out for burial," all this without any fear. We shall see later that this is a typical stupor content.

We will here include state 3 of Anna G. (See Chapter I, Case 1) who after the pronounced stupor was for two months merely dull, somewhat slowed and markedly apathetic. Although her orientation was not seriously affected, there was considerable interference with her intellectual processes, as shown in her wrong answers or her lack of answers when more difficult questions were asked.

A similar picture was presented in state 2 of Mary D. (See Chapter I, Case 4.) Here, to be sure, there were more marked stupor features in that the [48] patient wet and soiled, in addition to occasional spells when she lay with her head raised. But she spoke and acted fairly freely (even while soiling). By her replies she showed a considerable intellectual inefficiency, although, like Anna G., her orientation was not seriously disturbed. Here again there was complete affectlessness.

This gives us, therefore, five states which may be analyzed for the symptoms of partial stupor. The pictures of all five are unusually consistent. There is inactivity, marked but not complete; poverty of affect without perfect apathy; and a marked interference with the intellectual processes. The last can be studied better than in the deep stupors because these partial cases are more or less accessible to examination. There is a tendency for the patient to think much of death either in the onset or during the psychosis. Negativism seems much less prominent than in the deep stupors.

A natural criticism is that these cases merely had retarded depressions. Although this topic will be discussed fully in a later chapter, two differential characteristics should be mentioned now. First, depression is a highly emotional state in which the sadness of the patient is as evident from his facial and vocal expression as from what he says, while these stupor reactions are by observation and confession states of indifference. Secondly, there is no such disturbance of the intellectual processes in depression as is here chronicled. Let the retardation once be overcome so that the will is exercised and [49] no real defect is demonstrable. In our experience the cases of apparent depression with intellectual incapacity are found on closer study to be really stupors as other symptoms show.

[50]

CHAPTER III
SUICIDAL CASES

An important "catatonic" symptom is a tendency to sudden, impulsive, unexplainable acts. Such actions occur occasionally in benign stupors and, since we attempt an understanding of the reaction as a whole, an effort should be made to study these phenomena as well. The cases chosen showed persistent, quite affectless, yet very impulsive attempts at self-injury. They characterized the first of the three cases throughout, were present in one stage (the second) of the second patient, while in the last for one day there was behavior which can be similarly interpreted.

Mention has been made of the prominence, approaching universality, of the death idea in stupor. This is a subject to be discussed in length presently, but for the present we may say that there may be a delusion of death with dramatization of that state or a mere abandonment of the mental activities of life. It is but a step from corpselike behavior to suicidal attempts, psychologically speaking, yet this transition necessarily modifies the clinical picture, since one necessitates inactivity and the other activity. Secondarily, other atypical clinical features appear, as will be seen.

[51] Case 9.—*Pearl F.* Age: 24. Admitted to the Psychiatric Institute July 26, 1913.

F. H. A paternal aunt was insane. Both parents died long ago; the mother when the patient was a baby; the father when she was a girl. She came to this country when 17. In this country she had generally been a domestic. An older brother and sister were also in America.

P. H. She was described as sociable, good-natured, bright enough, not inclined to be depressed. She had little education. There was no former attack.

Four months before admission, the patient did not menstruate but was said not to have worried about this. A month later she began to show symptoms. She said she did not want to live, had done something wrong but could not or would not say what it was. Again she said a young man was going to sue her, a young Jewish fellow whom she had seen only a few times. She talked of turning on the gas. She also complained that people were looking at her and that the food was poisoned.

The patient after recovery gave the following version of the onset: She had a position on 99th St. for 2½ years. She liked the people there and often went to see them later. Her next position was in the Bronx. She was there for nine months. In the same house lived "Harry." After the work she used to talk to him in the yard and, after she left, she used to think of him and long for him. But she denied, with a very natural attitude, that she worried about him at the beginning of her psychosis. After the position in the Bronx she went to one on 96th St., where she was for four months. In the same house was a girl whom she liked and who was lively. When she left, the patient left too. This was a month before the psychosis began. When she left there, she got word that her employer on 99th St. had developed consumption and had to go out West, but did not worry over this news, she claimed. She looked for another position and had one for two weeks, but felt lonely, did not care to live. Then her sister took her to her home. She thought people were looking at her and were making remarks because she was not working. During this time she had a dream one night in which her dead mother appeared to her (in ordinary street clothes) and said to her that she (the patient) "was going away." She woke up [52] frightened. She was worried, thought she had not prayed enough for her mother, and asked her sister to pray also and to give money to the poor. She did not recall, or at any rate denied, speaking of the young man suing her.

She was then taken to a *private sanatorium*, where she was for two months preceding her admission to this hospital. There she was described as quiet, mute, tube-fed, resistive.

When well, the patient said that in this sanatorium she was first spoon-fed, cup-fed, later tube-fed, "I used to be scared of them, they used to put a spoon way down my throat and I had no appetite—I did not like them around me, they were mean to me. They used to let me stand without clothes, used to spite me." "If I did not want to dress myself, they used to hit me." "I used to feel lonesome for home and I imagined my people were there and that my sister passed the place without stopping." She was afraid of the nurses, thinking they wanted to kill her.

At the *Observation Pavilion* the patient was described as dull, but brightening up under examination. She made few spontaneous remarks, but in answer to questions said she was melancholy, tired of life, because she was in love with a Gentile fellow who refused to marry her. She also said "I get peculiar thoughts that I am going to die."

Under Observation: The patient's condition lasted for about two years. Much of the time she lay in bed, often with the covers pulled over her, sometimes with her legs drawn up, again in a more natural, comfortable position, or she sat up with her head bowed. She obeyed almost no commands. For months she soiled and wet herself, but never drooled. For a time she refused food consistently, lost flesh and had to be tube-fed. For the most part she said very little and, when one accosted her, she was apt to turn away. A few times, when further urged, she swore at the examiner. There was also persistent marked resistance towards any interference, sometimes merely passive or quite often, especially at first, with wriggling or severe scratching of her own body. There was often with this evidence of irritation or she moaned. Again she was described as quite affectless. One of the most striking features throughout a large part of the course were her suicidal attempts. She would try to strike her head against the iron bedpost, throw herself out of bed, throw herself [53] about generally, try to strangle herself with the sheets, try to pull out her tongue, all of which seemed to be done with great impulsiveness. Almost her only utterances had to do with death. She said she wanted to die, wanted to drop dead, did not want to live, wanted to kill herself, that she did not eat because she wanted to die. When once she was found tossing about and was asked whether she worried, she said "I know I am going to die." (You mean you will be killed?) "I don't care."

There were a few episodes which still have to be mentioned. Quite early in the course of the stupor, when she was restless, scratching herself and moaning, she once spoke quite freely. She said "Give me that fellow (Harry), I don't care, I can't help it. I must have him, even if it costs me my life." "I would feel happy if I could get him. O God, I love him—I will never get him even if I drop dead, I know I won't get him, the darling" (cries). (What if you did get him?) "I know I would lose him again." Then with shame she claimed she had had sexual relations with him (when well, denied). At the same interview, when the doctor sneezed, she said "Gesundheit." In June, 1914, she was seen smiling at times. But the first was the only episode when she spoke more freely, and the two occasions the only ones when she showed a frank affect.

The improvement commenced in April, 1915. Although still very inactive, she sometimes began to laugh and sing and talk a little to other patients. She also answered a few questions on April 22, 1915. Thus, when asked whether she wanted to go home, she said "No, I want to stay here." (Do you like it here?) "Yes" (smiles), "I can't get no other place; I have got to like it here." She smiled freely. To orientation questions, she knew the place, month, but not the year.

She continued inactive and above all diffident, but improved steadily and, when examined by the writer on November 15, she made a very natural impression and gave the retrospective account of the onset embodied in the history. She was quite frank, thanked the doctor for the interest he took in her case, and said for example, "You know I never thought I would get well. I quite gave up—I am very glad I am well now."

When questioned about her stay here, the patient evidently remembered much. She was able to say which wards she had [54] been in and approximately how long she had been in each one. She claimed that at first it "seemed strange." "I did not eat, I did not want to eat, I used to tell them to poison me and that I wanted to die, I was *disgusted*, I thought I would never go home." She also says she felt *angry*, wanted to kill herself. She bit and scratched "because I was nervous." She remembered talking about Harry, "I said I was in love with him, I thought I wanted to die because I could not have him." She also talked of having been *stubborn*. Sometimes she felt like running to the river. She also claimed she imagined people were false to her.

In one of the wards she said she thought people were there on her account, were waiting for her death. She did not care for a time whether she died or not. She knew she tried to choke herself occasionally. Asked how she behaved, she first said she was quiet. (Were you not restless?) "I used to get tired and have backache and roll around in bed." She also felt like running away sometimes, wanted to get out of bed and wanted to walk about. (What about going to the river?) "I used to say that." She claimed not to have been mixed up at any time and to remember everything. Remarkable is the fact that she claimed she *did not worry at all*, "*I felt I was lost and would not worry.* I used to worry at home and at Dr. M.'s (the private sanatorium) but not here. Here I never worried, I did not care where I went." She said she did not talk because she was bashful in the presence of doctors, sometimes she felt afraid of them, afraid they would kill her, put poison in her food when they fed her. "When my people came, I said I did not want to live, wanted to kill myself. I used to cry." Again asked why she did not talk, she admitted she really did not know. Once she said she was bashful because she soiled her bed. She did not want to go to the closet because she was afraid of the nurse. She denied hearing voices.

In addition to the activity incidental to her attempts at self-injury, this patient showed an unusual degree of resistiveness and with this some affect, for she appeared to be irritated and at times moaned. Still more unusual were the appearances [55] of delusions not associated with death but with a vivid form of life, namely, a love affair. Occasionally she spoke of her imaginary lover "Harry." Another atypical feature was a fair memory for the period when she was in stupor. She claimed to remember much of her movements and this claim was substantiated by her answers to questions after recovery.

Case 10. — *Margaret C.* Age: 23. Single. Admitted to the Psychiatric Institute November 13, 1913.

F. H. Heredity was absolutely denied. The mother is living and made a natural impression. The father died at 65, nine months before patient's admission, of cardio-renal disease. Two brothers and one sister died of acute diseases. One sister died in childbirth. Three brothers and one sister were said to be well.

P. H. The patient was bright and passed successfully through high school. For seven years prior to the psychosis she worked for the same company as clerk. She was described as efficient, conscientious, systematic, though sometimes upset by her work; as lively, talkative, cheerful, with somewhat of a temper and easily hurt, also as quite religious. She was more attached to her mother than to her father, but still more to her older sister, whose death precipitated her psychosis. She never had any love affair and was said not to have cared for men. Two months before admission, when her favorite sister was confined, the patient was quite worried about her, but relieved when she heard good news. A few hours later, however, the sister died suddenly. When the patient learned of the sister's death, she screamed, and screamed several times at the funeral. She did not cry, said she could not. After this she slept poorly, seemed nervous, went to church more, but there was no other change. She continued to work and, according to the employer, worked well.

Nine days before admission she would not get out of bed in the morning, said little and refused food. A few days later she was induced to take a walk, but she seemed to have no interest in anything. When she talked at all it was about her sister and [56] of wanting to go to a convent. When asked to do anything she said she would if it were God's will. She did not menstruate after her sister's death. When practically recovered, the patient attributed her breakdown to this tragedy. She added to the description above given that, soon after losing her sister, she had a fright at home. "It was the house in which my father died and one day when I was in bed I thought somebody came in." But she denied a vision and could not further explain.

At the *Observation Pavilion* she was very inactive, so that she had to be fed and cared for in every way, mute, often covering her head with a sheet, turning away when questioned and resistive when the physical examination was attempted. But at times she smiled or laughed.

Under Observation: 1. For two months the patient was generally inactive, sometimes lying in bed with her eyes tightly closed, or with her face covered by the sheets or buried in the pillow; or she sat inactive, staring, or with eyes closed, or her head buried in her arms. On one visit she had to be brought into the examining room in a wheel chair and lifted into another seat. A few times she was observed holding herself very tense with her head pressed against the end of the bed. But this inactivity was often interrupted by her going quickly into various rooms to kneel down, though she was never heard praying. Or she ran down the hall for no obvious reason. Or, again, she was found lying on the floor face down. She ate very poorly and had to be tube-fed a considerable part of the time. When this was done, she sometimes resisted severely, as she did in fact most nursing attentions. Thus she soon began to struggle when her hair was combed. She also resisted being taken to the toilet or being brought back. She did not soil or drool, however, but sometimes seemed to be in considerable distress before she finally literally ran to the closet. This resistance just spoken of consisted chiefly in making herself stiff and tense. Sometimes at the feeding she pulled up the cover when preparations were made and held to it tightly. Quite striking was the fact that with such resistance she sometimes, though by no means always, laughed loudly, as she did occasionally when she was talked to, or even without any external stimulation. This laughter always was one of genuine merriment and quite contagious, and by no means shallow or silly.

[57] Usually the patient was totally mute. The exceptions occurred mostly when her resistance was called forth. Thus one day when fed she said, "I wish you people would have more to do," or on another occasion, when she had resisted being brought into the examining room, she said, "I will get out of here if I break a leg." But once when the nurse accidentally tickled her, she said, "Since I am ticklish, I must be jealous — I should worry." She also answered very few questions and such responses as she made were chiefly expressions of resentment. Thus, when one kept urging her, she finally would say "stop," or after much urging "I am going to hurt you pretty quick." Sometimes she said "Go away," or "Let me alone." She was just as silent with the mother and the priest as with the physicians. On one occasion she told the nurse that the priest had told her to talk to the doctors, but that she had nothing to say. Sometimes she did not even look at the visitors, but turned away from them, as she did from the physicians, but at one visit from a priest, though she scarcely said anything, she held on to him when he was about to depart and would not let him go. Throughout this period, since scarcely any answers were given, nothing was known about her orientation, except when on admission she gave a few answers. She then thought she was at the Observation Pavilion, seemed unable to

tell even that the physician was a doctor, but knew the date. When asked how she came to Ward's Island, she said "By ambulance." The physical condition presented nothing of note, except for a certain sluggishness of the skin with marked comedones.

2. By *January*, 1914, the picture changed somewhat and she then presented the following state for an entire year: The mutism persisted and indeed became even more absolute, and she began to wet and soil constantly. This commenced as what seemed to be an act of spite as a part of her resistiveness, for the first time she soiled she seemed to do it deliberately when the nurses insisted that she allow them to put on a dress. Later this explanation no longer held. Tube-feeding too was for the most part necessary, the resistiveness continuing as before. But the inactivity was broken into much more than before by constant impulsive attempts to hurt herself in every conceivable way—by bumping her head against the wall, putting her head under the hot water faucet, trying to pound the leg of the bedstead on her [58] foot, striking herself, pinching her eyelids, pulling out her hair, trying to pick her radial artery, throwing herself out of bed, knocking her head against the bed rail, etc. This was done in silence but with what appeared a great determination that occasionally showed itself in her face. She also sometimes scowled and frowned. With the difficulty in feeding her and the constant impulsive excitement in which bruises could not always be avoided (once an extensive cellulitis developed in the arm which had to be lanced), the patient got weak, emaciated and exhausted; much of her hair fell out, although some she pulled out. It should be stated that during this entire impulsive state she could not be taken care of in the Institute ward, but was sent to a special ward in the Manhattan State Hospital, where suicidal patients are under constant watch. These impulsive attempts at self-injury lessened only towards the end of the period. Her laughter, which had been such a prominent trait, disappeared almost entirely during this entire phase. With all this, the general resistiveness, as has been stated, remained towards feeding or any other interference. It was only in the beginning associated with laughter as in the previous stage.

Although there were, as a rule, no spontaneous remarks and no replies, she on one occasion said spontaneously, probably referring to her unsuccessful attempts to kill herself: "I can't do it, I have no will." During the same period she once said: "I don't want to eat, I don't want to get well, I want to do penance and die."

By *January*, 1915 (i.e., a year after the second phase had commenced), she began to dress herself and eat, and also became clean. But she remained for the most part very inactive, sitting stolidly about all day and still without interest in her environment. The impulsive attempts at killing herself disappeared. Although she remained for months to come still inactive, she gradually began to talk a little, began to play a little on the piano, but said little to any one.

By *August*, 1915, she still was inactive, shy, standing about, or sitting picking her fingers, occasionally going to the piano, but evidently unable to finish anything. She had to be coaxed to come to the examining room and talked in a low tone. Often she commenced vaguely to speak and then stopped and could not [59] be made to repeat what she had been saying. Affectively she was remarkably frank, sometimes a little surly, or she showed a slight empty uneasiness. She could, however, be made to laugh heartily at times, or did so spontaneously on very slight provocation.

Some of her utterances were in harmony with her apparent indifference. It was difficult to get her to say how she felt even when thorough inquiries were made. Once she said, when asked about worrying, "I don't worry," or again "I get angry sometimes," or "I used to worry about my health, I don't now," or, when asked what her plans were, she said directly: "I don't care what happens." Again she said "I guess I am disagreeable," or "I guess I am a crank." Another interesting indication of her state was expressed in her repeated statement, "I don't know what I want." But she was oriented in a way, though not sure of her data. She would give most of her answers with a questioning inflection, "This is the Manhattan State Hospital, isn't it?" or she would say, "I don't know exactly where I am, it's Ward's Island, isn't it?" and in the same way she gave the day, date and year correctly. But she did not know the names of the physicians. At that time she could give many data about her family correctly, but was slow, even if correct, in calculation, and, though she got the gist of a test story, she left out some important details.

A retrospective account at that time showed she was uncertain about the Observation Pavilion, that she was not certain how she came to Ward's Island, "On a boat, I believe." It was clear that she did not remember the admission ward, about the Institute ward (in which she had been for the first two and a half months and in which she was again examined); she said it was familiar to her, but she was not certain that she had been in it. About the physician who saw most of her in these first two and a half months, she said that his voice seemed familiar, and she asked him whether he had tube-fed her (she had been tube-fed by him many times), but she again said, "No, you are not the one," and described as the man who had fed her the one who did it on the second ward where she was for a year. But she knew that she had been sent to the second ward, because she constantly tried to injure herself. These injuries she recalled but was unable [60] to say why she attempted them, "I suppose I didn't know what I was doing." She claimed she heard voices and had "all sorts" of imaginations, but could not be gotten to tell about them. When it was difficult for her to give an answer, she was apt to keep silent and then could be prodded without much success.

In *October*, 1915, there was further improvement, inasmuch as she began to converse some with other patients, played the piano and seemed able to carry a piece through. She was put in the occupation class and did quite well. At the interview with the physician she was still apt to laugh boisterously at slight provocation. Even now she had great difficulty in describing her condition and at the examination was often still quite vague. Thus, when asked how she felt, she said, "I do know I feel ridiculous—sometimes I feel kind of angry—I don't know—they say I am crazy but I am not, but I am hungry—I don't know whether I am or not, I don't know what I can do well," etc. This is quite characteristic. When asked whether she was worried, she said: "I don't know, am I worried?—yes, a little sometimes, I am to-day—I am so untidy—don't know what is the matter with me." Again: "Sometimes I lose my speech—I can't say what I feel, I don't know what it was." Later, half to herself: "I don't know what is the matter with me—I don't care anyway."

In *December*, 1915, there was still further improvement, and on the ward and in superficial conversation she made, towards the end of the month, in many ways a natural impression, though the laughter before described was still somewhat in evidence. It usually came not without occasion, but was, as a rule, quite out of proportion to the stimulus. She again said she could not explain why she tried to injure herself, claimed she did not feel it, and even claimed she did not remember doing it in the Institute but only in the second ward.

The defect in thinking which still remained is very difficult to formulate. She was now entirely oriented, no longer with any hesitation about the correctness of her information. She subtracted 7 from 100 very quickly and could from memory write a long poem, but there was a certain vagueness about her which partly may have been due to a still existing indifference. This vagueness consisted chiefly in a difficulty of attention or in her [61] capacity to grasp fully what was wanted. It is best illustrated by a few examples: After she had been asked about the *onset* of her sickness and she had said that what was on her mind then were prayers for the salvation of her relatives, she was asked exactly when it was that she thought of this; she answered "Now?" (What period were we talking of, the present or past?) "The present." (What did I ask you?) "About this period of my sickness." (Which one?) "What sickness?" She said herself at this point, "I am rather stupid" (quite placidly). Or again she said she did not know why she pounded her head, but finally said, "To get better and go home." (Do you think if you pounded your head against the wall you would go home sooner?) "I don't know—maybe." (How would it help you?) "You mean to go to the city?" (Yes.) "I don't know." Again when asked how her mind worked, she said, "Pretty quickly sometimes—I don't know." (As good as it used to?) "No, I don't think so." (What is the difference?) This had to be repeated several times, at which she said, "There is no difference." (What did I ask you?) "The difference." (The difference between what?) "You did not say." Equally striking was the fact that when she was jokingly told "If it snows to-night, we shall have a black Christmas," she did not grasp the absurdity at once, but in a rather puzzled way asked, "Why?"

She was then discharged on parole, two years and one month after admission. Soon after discharge her menstruation, which had been absent throughout her psychosis, returned. On her discharge she had regained her normal weight, and during the two subsequent months gained fifteen pounds.

She then recovered completely, so that three months after discharge she made a very natural impression. She said, on looking back over her state with impulsive excitement, that she constantly had the idea that she wanted to punish herself, but that *she did not know why*, and did not think she was sad or worried.

Considering only the second phase of the psychosis, this deep stupor showed many interruptions, due not merely to her suicidal efforts but also to her resistiveness. The condition, too, was not so com [62] pletely affectless as one expects a deep stupor to be. In the first stage there was much sudden laughter, reminding one of dementia præcox (except for its never being shallow or silly) and this persisted into the first part of the second phase. The actual attempts at self-injury brought out emotion, for with them she scowled and frowned as well as showing considerable energy.

To these may be added the following case. It is not unlike the ordinary stupor in the fact that there was intense inactivity and mutism with great tenseness. The remarkable trait was, however, that for a whole day she forcibly held her breath until she got blue in the face. The case in detail is as follows:

Case 11.—*Rosie K.* Age: 18. Admitted to the Psychiatric Institute January 24, 1907.

F. H. Both parents were living. The father was a loafer. Nine brothers and sisters were said to be well, with the exceptions of one brother who had an irritable temper, and of a markedly inferior sister.

P. H. The patient was a Galician Hebrew, a shirtwaist operator. Not much was known about her make-up, but it is certain that she was a bright girl. The patient herself said after recovery that her father was nagging her constantly with complaints that she was not making enough money, although he himself did not work and she contributed much to the support of her family. She disliked him very much and claimed that all her relatives worried her, except her mother.

Nine weeks before admission a messenger came into the shop where she worked and said, "Rosie, your father is dead" (the message was intended for a fellow worker). In spite of the fact that the matter was explained, she was upset and nervous enough to be taken home. Though she continued to work for over two weeks, she worried over many trivial matters and talked [63] much about this. She also said that everything looked queer at her home and complained of having difficulty in concentrating her mind. Finally she became elated and talkative. Nothing is known of any special ideas.

At the *Observation Pavilion* she appeared to be typically manic.

Then she was sent to an institution where she remained for six weeks. The report from there stated that she was for ten days "elated, excited, talkative, with flight of ideas." Then her condition suddenly changed to a marked reduction of activity, in which she neither spoke spontaneously nor answered questions. She "appeared to sleep," but was said to have talked to her people. When interfered with, she was resistive and sometimes let herself fall out of bed. On the other hand, she occasionally wandered about at night. It should be added that during the stupor an alveolar abscess developed which discharged pus. It was washed out and healed.

Then she was sent to the Manhattan State Hospital and admitted to the service of the Psychiatric Institute.

Under Observation: 1. On the first day she lay in bed with cyanotic extremities, weak pulse, grunting, moaning and not responding in any way when examined. After this the moaning and grunting ceased and she was essentially indifferent, and for the most part kept her eyes closed. Often she wet and soiled herself. She was resistive to any care or examination. She would not eat, as a rule, but again gulped down milk offered her. For a considerable time she had to be tube-fed. During the early part of this stupor she once took a paper from the doctor, examined it, and then gave it back without saying anything, or again she peered around silently, or asked to go home, or again, on a few occasions, answered a question or two or spoke some unintelligible words. Orientation could not be established.

2. After a few weeks she became more rigid, a condition which continued for six months. She let saliva collect in her mouth, and drooled. She had to be tube-fed. She lay very rigid, with very pronounced general tension, with her lips puckered, hands clenched, sometimes holding her eyes tightly closed, and often with marked

perspiration. For one day she held her breath until she was blue in the face. On the same day she was extremely [64] rigid, so that she could be raised by her head with only her heels resting on the bed. Her eyes were tightly shut and she was in profuse perspiration. Sometimes she interrupted this by a deep breath, only again to resume the forcible holding of her breath. On another day towards the end of the period, while quite stiff, she kept grunting and screaming "murder." The soiling continued. She never spoke.

Physical condition during the stupor: At first she had a coated tongue, foul breath and a fetid diarrhea. The latter was treated with high colonic flushing and mild diet. Urine normal—gynecologically normal. General neurological and physical examination not possible. At the same time she had for two weeks a temperature which often reached 100° or a little above, a weak, irregular but not rapid pulse, a leucocytosis of 17,500 and 80% hemoglobin. When she began to refuse food and before she was tube-fed regularly, she twice had syncopal attacks and lost considerable flesh which was gradually regained under tube-feeding. After the diarrhea she was habitually constipated. Cyanosis of the extremities seemed to have been present only at first.

3. Six months after admission she began to make very free facial movements—winking, raising the eyebrows—and soon developed an excitement with marked elation. She had to be kept in the continuous bath, talked continuously, whistled, sang, was markedly erotic towards the physician, careless in exposing herself and often obscene in her talk. Most of her productions were determined by the environment. She was therefore quite distractible, very alert; sometimes she was meddlesome, again irritable, irascible. The following illustrates her productions: "Send for my husband, S.—He had one sister as big as that. She likes candy.... My father is underneath and my mother is on top because she is fat and he is skinny.... Wait till the sun shines, Nellie—we will be happy, Nellie—don't you sigh, sweetheart, you and I—wait till the sun shines by and by.... Come in (as noise is heard)—I bet that is my husband—my name is Regina K. (mother's name)—my mother's name is the same—I got a little sister named Regina—she is my husband." When she heard the word pain, she said, "Who says paint, Pauline used paint, I used paint," etc.

[65] Towards the end of August she had pneumonia, which did not change her condition.

By October she was well, having gradually settled down. She had good insight.

Retrospectively: She laid very little stress on the false report of the father's death. She claimed to remember being at the Observation Pavilion, but to recall very little of the other hospital. Unfortunately an inquiry was not made regarding her memory during the stupor period under observation with the exception of the fact that she said she wanted to die and therefore refused food.

She was seen in March, 1913, appeared perfectly well, and stated she had been well during the entire interval.

If this forced holding of the breath had been the only anomaly, one would, perhaps, not be justified in drawing any conclusions as to its significance. But the deep stupor was interrupted again for a day by grunting and screaming of "murder." This is certainly indicative of a compulsive death idea and retrospectively she spoke of having refused food in order to die. The latter seems to indicate some connection between her negativism and death. Consequently, even if we regard the breath holding as resistiveness, it would still be related to her idea of dissolution. Her negativism went beyond ordinary limits in that it affected the expression of the face.

When we consider these three cases together, we see that what would otherwise have been deep stupors with profound inactivity, were modified by activity in two directions: suicidal and resistive. Presuming that the symptoms of stupor are all interrelated, we can see a reason why the affect should [66] also have been altered. When one is modified, this should influence the other. When the activity is increased, the emotional concomitants of impulsive acts tend to break through as well. Hence the changes observed in these cases in facial expression and tone of voice. It is noteworthy, too, that all three showed a tendency for laughter to appear, as if, the emotions once stirred, it was possible for them to be exhibited in other than unpleasant forms. So, too, it was possible for ideas unrelated to the stupor picture, such as those of lovers, to occur sporadically. Finally, since activity must imply some contact with environment, the first of these cases at least showed less interference with the intelligence than is usual. In general, one may conclude that any aberration from the pure type of stupor tends to allow other impurities to appear.

[67]

CHAPTER IV
THE INTERFERENCES WITH THE INTELLECTUAL PROCESSES

This is one of the most interesting and important of the stupor symptoms. We are accustomed to think of the functional psychoses having symptoms to do with emotions and ideas in the main, and, conversely, that disorientation, etc., observed in such cases is merely the result of distraction, poor attention or coöperation. But in stupor the deficit in understanding, incapacity to solve simple problems and failure of memory seem deep-rooted and fundamental symptoms. So far is this true that Bleuler [5] looks on "schizophrenic" cases with this symptom of "Benommenheit" as organic in etiology. It may be said at the outset that we do not share this view for many reasons. One at least may now be stated as it seems to be final. In benign stupor purely mental stimuli may change the whole clinical picture abruptly and with this produce a change in the intellectual functioning such as we never see in organic dementias or clouded states. We find it more satisfactory to attempt a correlation of this with the other symptoms on a purely functional basis, as will be explained later.

[68] For the study of the interferences with the intellectual processes during stupor reaction, we have two sources of information: The first is derived from the account which the patient is able to give in regard to what he remembers as having taken place around him or in his mind during the stupor period; the second is the direct observation of partial stupor reactions.

1. Information Derived from the Patient's Retrospective Account

We will start with the cases of marked stupor mentioned in Chapter I. Anna G.'s (Case 1) psychosis commenced at home, and under observation lasted with great intensity for five months. She remembered only vaguely the carriage going to the Observation Pavilion, had no recollection of the latter, nor of her transfer to the Manhattan State Hospital and of most of the stay at the Institute ward, including the tube- or spoon-feeding which had to be carried on for four months. She also claimed that she did not know where she was until four or five months after admission. She was amnesic for her delusions and hallucinations. Of Caroline DeS. (Case 2) we have no information. Of Mary F. (Case 3), whose stupor began at home and under observation lasted two years, we find that she had no recollection of coming to the hospital, what ward she came to, who the doctor and nurses were (with whom she became acquainted later), in fact she [69] claimed that for about a year she did not know where she was. But she remembered having been tube-fed (this took place over a long period). Mary D.'s (Case 4) stupor also commenced at home, and under observation lasted for three months. She had no recollection of going to the Observation Pavilion, of the transfer to Manhattan State Hospital, and of a considerable part of her stay here, including such obtrusive facts as a presentation before a staff meeting, an extensive physical and a blood examination, and she claimed not to have known for a long time where she was. Annie K.'s (Case 5) stupor commenced at home. Although she recalled the last days there and some ideas and events at the Observation Pavilion, the memory of the journey to Ward's Island was vague, as was that of entrance to the ward, and she claimed not to have known where she was for quite a while. Specific occurrences, such as the taking of her picture (with open eyes two months after admission), an examination in a special room, her own mixed-up writing (end of second week) were not remembered. But it is quite interesting that an angry outburst of another patient within this same period, which was evidently not recorded, is clearly remembered.

We shall later show that when the patient comes out of a stupor the condition may be such that, for a time at least, retrospective accounts are difficult to obtain. It must also be remembered that not infrequently the more marked stupors may be followed by milder states, and it is important, if we [70] wish to determine how much is remembered, not to confuse the two states or not to let the patient confuse them. For example, Mary D. (Case 4), who showed two separate phases, while she claimed not to know of many external facts, also added that she could not understand the questions which were asked. From observation in other cases it seems that in marked stupor any such recollection about the patient's own mental processes would be quite inconsistent. We have to assume, therefore, that this remark referred in reality to the second milder phase, for which, as we shall see, it is indeed quite characteristic. It is not necessary to burden the reader with other cases, all of which consistently gave such accounts.

We see, then, that in the marked stupor the intellectual processes are regularly interfered with, as evidenced by almost complete amnesia for external events and internal thoughts. In other words, this would indicate that the minds of these patients were blank. Inasmuch as direct observation during the stupor adduces little proof of mentation, we may assume that such mental processes as may exist in deepest stupor are of a primitive, larval order.

Before we examine more carefully the milder grades of stupor, it will be necessary to say a few words about the retrospective account which the patient gives of intellectual difficulties during the incubation period of the psychosis. As a matter of fact, we find that these accounts are remarkably uniform. While some patients, to be sure, speak of [71] a more or less sudden lack of interest or ambition which came over them, others of them speak plainly of a sudden mental loss. Mary. C. (Case 7) claimed she suddenly got mixed up and lost her memory. Laura A. spoke at any rate of suddenly having felt dazed and stunned. Mary D. (Case 4) said she felt she was losing her mind and that she could not understand what she was reading. Maggie H. (Case 14) began to say that her head was getting queer. We see from this that the interferences with the intellectual processes may in the beginning be quite sudden.

In some instances a more detailed retrospective account was taken, which may throw some light upon the interferences with the intellectual processes with which we are now concerned. Emma K., whose case need not be taken up in detail, had a typical marked stupor which lasted for nine months, preceded by a bewildered, restless, resistive state for five days. She was in the Institute ward for the first four months, including the five days above mentioned; later in another ward. When asked what was the first ward which she remembered, she mentioned the one after the Institute ward, and when asked who the first physician was, she mentioned the one in charge of the second ward. However, when taken to the Institute ward, she said it looked familiar, and was able to point to the bed in which she lay, though somewhat tentatively. The same rousing of memory occurred when the first physician, who saw her daily, was pointed out to her. She remembered having [72] seen him, and then even recalled the fact that he had thrown a light into her eyes, but remembered nothing else. This observation would seem to show that with some often repeated or very marked mental stimuli (throwing electric light into her eyes) a vague impression may be left, so that it may at least be possible to bring about a recollection with assistance, whereas spontaneous memory is impossible. In another instance, the patient was confronted with a physician who had seen a good deal of her. She said that he looked familiar to her, but she was unable to say where she had seen him. Here then again evidence that a certain vague impression was made by a repeated stimulus.

Another feature should here be mentioned, namely, that isolated facts may be remembered when the rest is blank. We have seen above that Annie K. (Case 5), while very vague about most occurrences, recalled a sudden angry outburst in detail. Another patient, though the period of the stupor was a blank, recalled some visits of her mother. At these times, as she claimed, she thought she was to be electrocuted and told her mother so, "Then it would drop out of my mind again." These facts are very interesting. We can scarcely account for such phenomena in any other way than by assuming that certain influences may temporarily lift the patient out of the deepest stupor. In spite of the fact that stupors often last for one or two years almost without change, a fact which would argue that the stupor reaction is a remarkably set, stable state, [73] we see in sudden episodes of elation that this is not the case, and other experiences point in the same direction. A similar observation was made on a case of typical stupor with marked reduction of activity and dullness. A rather cumbersome electrical apparatus (for the purpose of getting a good light for pupil examination) was brought to her bedside. Whereas before, she had been totally unresponsive, she suddenly wakened up, asked whether "those things" would blow up the place, and whether she was to be electrocuted. During this anxious state she responded promptly to commands, but after a short time relapsed into her totally inactive condition. We have, of course, similar experiences when we try to get stuporous patients to eat, who, after much coaxing may, for a short time, be made to feed themselves, only to relapse into the state of inactivity.

Such variations are paralleled, as we shall later show, by a suddenly pronounced deepening of the thinking disorder. We have already seen that the onset may be quite sudden. All this indicates that, in spite of a certain stability, sudden changes are not uncommon. Finally, we know that, in spite of the fact that stupor is an essentially affectless reaction, certain influences may produce smiles or tears, or, above all, angry outbursts, which again can hardly be interpreted otherwise than by assuming that those influences have temporarily produced a change in the clinical picture, in the sense of lifting the patient out of the depth of the stupor. All these [74] facts suggest that inconsistencies in recollection are correlated with changes in the clinical picture.

As is to be expected, the cases with partial stupors remember much more of what externally and internally happened during their psychoses. Rose Sch. (Case 6), who had a partial stupor during which she answered questions but showed a great difficulty in thinking, said retrospectively that she felt mixed up and could not remember. Although she recalled with details the Observation Pavilion and her transfer, she was not clear about their time relations (how long in the Observation Pavilion, how long in the first ward). Mary C. (Case 7), whose activity was not entirely interfered with and who showed some thinking disorder, said retrospectively that she could not take in things. Henrietta H. (Case 8), who had a partial stupor, claimed to have known all along where she was, but that she felt mixed up, that her thoughts wandered and that she felt confused about people. In the cases where a partial stupor was preceded by a marked one, such as in phase 2 of Anna G. (Case 1) and phase 2 of Mary D. (Case 4), we have no retrospective account regarding the partial stupor, because emphasis in the analysis was naturally laid on the period comprising the most marked disorder. However, we can gather from the few cases at our disposal that the patients retrospectively lay stress chiefly on their inability to understand the situation.

We finally have to consider the group of suicidal cases. We have information only in regard to two [75] cases, namely, Margaret C. (Case 10) and Pearl F. (Case 9). In both of these, we find that a good many things that happened during the period under consideration were remembered, as were also the patients' own actions. In Rosie K. (Case 11) we have at least the evidence that she remembered her own impulses, namely, that she refused food because she wanted to die. In other words, in these partial stupors with impulsive suicidal tendencies the interference with the intellectual processes seems to be moderate, and memory for external events not markedly affected.

2. Information Derived from Direct Observation

The evidence can best be presented by considering the details of some cases.

Rose Sch. (Case 6) was remarkable, in connection with the present problem, in her unusually poor answers. She either merely repeated the questions, or made irrelevant superficial replies, or said she did not know, this even with very simple questions. When better, too, though not quite well, she showed striking discrepancies in time relations and incapacity to correct them. It would seem that in this case there was something more than an acute interference with the intellectual processes, such as we are here discussing. As a matter of fact, we have the statement in the history that the patient herself said she was slow at learning in school and had not much of an education. A congenital intellectual defect [76] and the attitude which it creates may, however, as my experience has repeatedly shown me, very greatly exaggerate an acute thinking disorder. The case, therefore, while it shows us an unquestionably acute interference with the intellectual processes, does not give us useful information about its nature. More information can be gathered from Mary D. (Case 4). Even toward the end of her marked stupor some replies were obtained chiefly by making her write. When asked to write Manhattan State Hospital, she wrote Manhatt Hhospshosh, and for Ward's Island, Ww. Iland. Again, instead of writing 90th Street, she wrote 90theath Street. These are plainly reactions of the path of least resistance or, in these instances, of perseveration. Of the same nature are some of her other replies in writing or speaking.

After she had been asked to write her name, she was requested to add her address, or the name of the hospital; she merely repeated the name. Similarly, when asked whether she knew the examiner, she said "Yes," but when urged to give his name, she gave her own. In the partial stupor at a time when she knew where she was, knew the names of some people about her, the year and approximately the date, she made mistakes in calculation and could not get the point of a test story. Moreover, she failed in retention tests without there being any evidence of anything like a marked fundamental retention disorder, such as we find in Korsakoff psychosis. It seems that these results are best termed defects in attention, which chiefly interfere [77] with the apprehension of more difficult tasks. As we shall see later, this seems to be rather characteristic of these cases. Another point which should be mentioned is the fact that her reaction to questions which she was unable to answer (such as matters which referred to her amnesic periods) was peculiar, inasmuch as she did not only not try to think them out, but seemed indifferent to her incapacity, simply leaving the question unanswered. This too, as we shall see later, is characteristic. Laura A., at a time when she could be made to reply, merely repeated the question, again a reaction of least resistance. The same patient sometimes asked, "Where am I?" Mary C. (Case 7) made similar queries. Although she was at times approximately oriented, she would say, "I don't know where I am," or "I can't realize where I am," or more pointedly, "I can't take in my surroundings." She often did not answer and sometimes seemed bewildered by the questions. Henrietta H. (Case 8) again showed some defect of orientation and mistakes in calculation, and above all, marked mistakes in writing (for Manhattan State Hospital—Manhaton Hotspal). A special feature here is that this occurred immediately after she had been quite talkative, but suddenly had relapsed into a dull state. Anna G. (Case 1), during the third phase of her psychosis, showed the following: Although she was approximately oriented and answered promptly simple questions; e.g., about orientation or simple calculation, she, like these other patients, simply remained silent when more [78] difficult intellectual tasks were required of her (more difficult calculations); or when she was asked how long she had been here (which involved data that could not be available to her, owing to her amnesia); or when questions were put to her regarding her feelings or the condition she had passed through. On the other hand, she sometimes gave appropriate replies in the words "yes" or "no," but it was difficult to say whether these answers did not also represent the path of least resistance.

We will finally take up the last phase of Margaret C. (Case 10). Although she was entirely oriented, there was a certain vagueness about her answers which is difficult to formulate. She was telling about the onset of her sickness and said that at that time her mind was taken up with prayers about the salvation of her relatives. She was asked exactly when it was that she thought of this and she answered "Now?" (What period are we talking about?) "The present." (What did I ask you?) "About this period of my sickness." (Which one?) "What sickness?" She said herself at this point, "I am rather stupid." Again when asked how her mind worked, she said, "Pretty quickly sometimes—I don't know." (As good as it used to?) "No, I don't think so." (What is the difference?) "There is no difference." (What did I ask you?) "The difference." (The difference between what?) "You did not say." In this the shallowness of her comprehension and thinking is well shown, and it seems here again perhaps justifiable to formulate the main [79] defect as one of attention, which prevents completion of a complicated process of comprehension. A feature of further interest in this case is that automatic intellectual processes, such as those necessary for the writing of a long poem from memory, were not interfered with.

Summary

In the most pronounced stupor we have evidently a more or less complete standstill in thinking processes. Practically no impressions are registered and consequently nothing is remembered except events that occurred in some short periods when some affective stimulus, or a brief burst of elation, lifts the patient temporarily out of the deep stupor. It is impossible to say whether the statement of a complete standstill has to be qualified. In some stupors repeated environmental stimuli sometimes make at least a vague impression, so that while spontaneous recollection is impossible a feeling of familiarity is present when the patient is again confronted with this environment. This might be an exception to the dictum of complete mental vacuity, or it may be that there are somewhat less pronounced stupor reactions. When more is perceived, there is often a retrospective statement of having felt mixed up, being unable to take in things, or, directly under observation, the patient may say, "I cannot realize where I am," "I cannot take in my surroundings." In harmony with this is the fact that questions often produce a certain bewilderment. [80] In quite pronounced states in which some replies can still be obtained, we find that the intellectual processes may be interfered with to the extent of a paragraphia, i.e., a remarkably mixed-up writing in which perseveration (one form of following the path of least resistance) plays a prominent part. This same principle is also seen in such reactions as the repetition of the question or the senseless repetition of a former answer. These phenomena remind us of what we see in epileptic confusions, in epileptic deterioration and in arteriosclerotic dementia.

In milder cases difficulties in orientation may be more or less marked; or there may be incapacity to think out problems, although the orientation is perfect. The more automatic mental processes may run smoothly (memory and calculation may be excellent) and there may yet be a certain shallowness in thinking, a defect of attention (a purely descriptive term) which is most obvious in the patient's inability to grasp clearly the drift of what is going on or the meaning of complicated questions. I am inclined to think that poor results in retention tests are entirely due to this attention disorder, for we have no evidence of any fundamental retention defect such as we find in the totally different organic stupors. From a practical point of view it is important at this place to call attention to the fact that such mild changes are particularly seen in end stages. Even when pronounced negativistic tendencies do not play a prominent rôle, the patient is then apt to be silent chiefly as a result of the residual [81] disorder in the intellectual processes. Still more striking are the conditions which are on a somewhat higher level and in which the shallowness of the responses, due to the residual disorder of attention, together with the last traces of the affectlessness, are apt to create the impression of a dementia. In such cases the opinion is often held that the patient has reached a defect stage from which recovery is impossible, whereas a thorough knowledge of these end stages teaches us that they are not only recoverable but quite typical for the terminal phases of stupor.

Considering these data, especially those gathered in the end stages, it would appear that there is no tendency in this intellectual disorder associated with the stupor reaction for any special side of mental activity to be most prominently affected. It looks rather as if it were a question of a general diminution of the capacity to make a mental effort which in its different intensities accounts for the symptoms.

Footnotes:

[5] See Chapter XV.

CHAPTER V
THE IDEATIONAL CONTENT OF THE STUPOR

Brief survey of the ideas associated with stupor: Having thus described the formal manifestations of the various stupor reactions, it will now be interesting to see what ideas seem to be associated with these reactions. It is, of course, impossible to obtain during a considerable part of the stupor any statement of the patients' thoughts. We therefore have to depend on their utterances during periods when the inactivity temporarily ceases, or on the retrospective account which the patient gives after the stupor has completely disappeared; and as we shall see, we also may obtain considerable information by studying the ideas which occur in the period preceding the stupor. These last may be autogenous delusions or thoughts about actual events which precipitated the psychosis.

It is not likely that many observers have a very clear conception about what sort of ideas to expect. We have, as a rule, not been in the habit of paying much attention to the content of delusions, hallucinations, and the like. So far as we could judge, therefore, the ideas expressed might be expected to be fairly multiform, and it was distinctly interesting [83] to us when we found a marked tendency for the trends of ideas to remain within a certain small compass. [6] It was possible, to state this at once, to show that in by far the majority of cases the same set of ideas returned, and that these ideas had among themselves a definite inner relationship, being concerned with thoughts of "death." In isolated instances other ideas were found as well, and they will have to be discussed later. For the present we shall take up more habitual content.

In addition to the eleven cases already described, it may be well to cite four others which present material now of interest to us.

Case 12.—*Charlotte W.* Age: 30. Admitted to the Psychiatric Institute October 21, 1905.

F. H. The father was alcoholic and quick-tempered; he died when the patient was a child. The mother was alcoholic and was insane at 40 (a state of excitement from which she recovered). A brother had an attack of insanity in 1915. A maternal uncle died insane.

P. H. The patient was described as jolly, having many friends. She got on well in school and was efficient at her work.

She was married at 23 and got on well with her husband. The latter stated, however, that she masturbated during the first year of her married life. The first child was born without trouble.

First Attack at 25: Two or three days after giving birth to a second child, her mother burst into the room intoxicated. The patient immediately became much frightened, nervous, and developed a depressive condition with crying, slowness and inability to do things. During this state she spoke of being bad and told [84] her husband that a man had tried to have intercourse with her before marriage. This attack lasted six months and ended with recovery.

When 29, a year before her admission, she had an abortion performed, and four months later another. Her husband was against this, but she persisted in her intention. Seven months before admission she went to the priest, confessed and was reproved. It is not clear how she took this reproof, but at any rate no symptoms appeared until three weeks later, after burglars had broken into a nearby church. Then she became unduly frightened, would not stay at home, said she was afraid the burglars would come again and kill "some one in the house." The patient herself stated later, during a faultfinding period, that at that time she was afraid somebody would take her honor away, and that she thought burglars had taken her "wedding dress." "Then," she added, "I thought I would run away and lead a bad life, but I did not want to bring disgrace to the family."

The general condition which she presented at this time is described as one of apprehensiveness when at home. For this reason she was for five weeks (it is not clear exactly at what period) sent to her sister, where she was better. About a month before the patient was admitted, the husband moved, whereupon she got depressed, complained of inability to apply herself to work, became slow and inactive, and blamed herself for having had the abortion performed. She began to speak of suicide and was committed because she bought carbolic acid. She later said that while in the *Observation Pavilion* she imagined her children were cut up.

Under Observation the condition was as follows:

1. For the first three days the patient, though for the most part not showing any marked mood reaction, was inclined at times to cry, and at such times complained essentially that this was a terrible place for a person who was not insane.

2. On the fourth day the condition changed, and it will be advisable to describe her state in the form of abstracts of each day.

On *October 24* the patient began to be preoccupied and to answer slowly. A few days later she became distinctly dull, walked about in an indifferent way or lay in bed immobile. [85] Twice on *October 27* she said in a low tone and with slight distress, "Give me one more chance, let me go to him." But she would not answer questions. At times she lapsed into complete immobility, lying on her back and staring at the ceiling. When the husband came in the afternoon, she clung to him and said: "Say good-by forever, O my God, save me." Again, very slowly with long pauses and with moaning, she said: "You are going to put me in a big hole where I will stay for the rest of my life." On *October 28* she was found with depressed expression and spoke in a rather low tone, but not with decided slowness as had been the case on the day before. She pleaded about having her soul saved; "Don't kill me"; "Make me true to my husband"; once, "I have confessed to the wrong man the shame of my life." Later she said she did not tell the truth about her life before marriage. Again she wanted to be saved from the electric chair. At times she showed a tendency to stare into space and to leave questions unanswered.

3. From now on a more definite stupor occurred, which is also best described in summaries of the individual notes.

Oct. 29. Lies in bed with fixed gaze, pointing upward with her finger and is very resistive towards any interference. She has to be catheterized.

Oct. 30. Can be spoon-fed but is still catheterized. During the morning she knelt by the bed and would not answer. At the visit she was found in a rather natural position, smiling as the physician approached, saying "I don't know how long I have been here." Then she looked out of the window fixedly. At first she did not answer, but, when the physician asked whether she knew his name, she laughed and said, "I know your name—I know my name." Then she would not answer any more questions but remained immobile, with fixed gaze. When her going home was mentioned, however, she flushed and tears ran down her cheek, though no change in the fixedness of her attitude or in her facial expression was seen.

Nov. 1. Lies flat on her back with her hands elevated. She is markedly resistive.

Nov. 2. Free from muscular tension and more responsive. When asked whether she felt like talking, she said in a whining tone, "No, go away—I have to go through enough." Then she [86] spoke of not knowing how long the nights and days were, of not having known which way she was going. When asked who the physician was she whimpered and said, "You came to tell me what was right." She called him "Christ" and another physician "Jim" (husband's name), though, later in the interview, she gave their correct names. When asked about the name of another physician, she said: "He looks like my cousin, he was here, they all came the first night. I did not take notice who it was till I went through these spirits, then I knew it was right."—She paused and added: "My God—mother it was; she is here on Earth, somewhere in a convent—Sister C. (who actually is in a convent) she was here, too, I could hear her." She said they all came to try to save her. When asked whether she had been asleep, she said: "No, I wasn't asleep, I was mesmerized, but I am awake now—sometimes I thought I was dead." (When?) "The time I was going to Heaven." Again: "I went to Heaven in spirit, I came back again—the wedding ring kept me on Earth—I will have to be crucified now." (Tell me about it.) "Jim will have to pick my eyes out—I think it is him. Oh, it is my little girl." (Who told you?) "The spirits told me." Again: "Little birds my children—I can't see them any more—I must stay here till I die." (Why?) "The spirits told me—till I pick every one of my eyes out and my brains too." When asked what day it was, she said, "It must be Good Friday." (Why?) "Because God told me I must die on the cross as he did." When asked why she had not spoken the day before, she said that "Jesus Christ in Heaven" had told her she should not tell anything, "till all of you had gone, then I could go home with him, because that is the way we came in and it was Jim too all the time." Finally she said crossly, "Go away now, you are all trying to keep me from Jim" (crying).

Nov. 3. Knelt by bed during the night. This morning lies in bed staring, resistive, again she is markedly cataleptic. She has to be spoon-fed, and is totally unresponsive. In the afternoon she was found staring and resistive. Presently she said with tears: "I am waiting to be put on the cross."

Nov. 4. Still has to be catheterized. She sits up, staring, with expressionless face, but when asked how she felt she responded and said feebly: "I don't know how I feel or how I [87] look or how long I have been here or anything." (What is wrong?) "Oh, I only want to go to a convent the rest of my days." (Why?) "Oh, I have only said wrong things, I thought I would be better dead, I could not do anything right." Later she again began to stare.

Nov. 5. During the night she is said to have been restless and wanted to go to church. To-day she is found staring, but not resistive. When questioned she sometimes does not answer. She said to the physician, "I should have gone up to Heaven to you and not brought me down here." She called the physician "Uncle James." Again she said, "I want to go up to see Jim." Sometimes she looks indifferent, again somewhat bewildered.

Nov. 6. She eats better, catheterizing is no longer necessary. She is found lying in bed, rigid, staring, resistive, does not answer at first, later appears somewhat distressed, says "I want to go and see Jim." (Where?) "In Heaven." She gave the name of the place and of the physician, also the date.

Nov. 8. In the forenoon, after she had presented a rather immobile expression and had answered a few orientation questions correctly, she suddenly beckoned into space, then shook her fist in a threatening manner. When later asked about this, she said: "Jim was down there and I wanted to get him in." (And?) "You was up here first." (And?) "I thought we was going down down, up up—the boat— — you came in here for—to lock Jim out so we wouldn't let him in." Later she said, when asked whether anything worried her, "Yes, you are taking Jim's place."

Nov. 9. During the night she is reported to have varied between stiffness with mutism and a more relaxed state. Once, the nurse found her with tears, saying "I want to go down the hall to my sister—to the river," and a short time later with fright: "Is that my mother?" Again she said: "Oh dear, I wish this boat would stop—stop it—where are we going?" In the forenoon she was quiet and unresponsive. In the afternoon she said in a somewhat perplexed way, "We were in a ship and we were 'most drowned." (When was that?) "Day before yesterday it must have been"—Again she said in the same manner: "It was like water. I was going down. I could hear a lot of things." She claimed this happened "to-day." "I saw all the people in [88] here, it was all full of water," "I have been lying here a long time—do you remember the time I was under the ground and it seemed full of water and every one got drowned and a sharp thing struck me?" "I was out in a ship and I went down there in a coffin." When asked whether she had been frightened at such times, she said: "No, I didn't seem to be, I just lay there." She also said: "the water rushed in," and when asked why she put up her arms, she said, "I did it to save the ship."

Nov. 10. She is still fairly free. She said that when she was on the ship things looked changed, "the picture over there looked like a saint, the beds looked queer." (How do things look now?) "All right." (The picture too?) "The same as when I was going down into a dark hole." When asked later in the day where she was, she said, "In the Pope's house, Uncle Edward is it?" but after a short time she added, "It is Ward's Island, isn't it?"

Nov. 11. Inactive, inaccessible, but for the most part not rigid.

Nov. 14. Varies between mutism with resistance and more relaxed inactivity. To-day lies in a position repeatedly assumed by her, namely, on her stomach with head raised, resistive towards any interference, immobile face, totally inaccessible.

Nov. 15. Freer. She said: "One day I was in a coffin, that's the day I went to Heaven." She also said she used to see "the crucifix hanging there" (on the ceiling)—"not now but when I was going to Heaven." (When was that?) "Over in that bed" (her former bed). Later she added, "The place changed so ... things used to be coming up and down (dreamily)—that was the day I was coming up on the ship or going down." She is quite oriented.

Nov. 17. Usually stands about with immobile face, preoccupied, but she eats voluntarily.

Nov. 24. When the husband and sister came a few days ago she said she was glad to see them, embraced them, cried and is said to have spoken quite freely. To-day she speaks more freely than usually. When asked why she had answered so little, she said she could not bring herself to say anything, though she added spontaneously, "I knew what was said to me." When shown a picture of her cataleptic attitude with hands raised, she [89] said dreamily, "I guess that must have been the day I went to Heaven, everything seemed strange, things seemed to be going up and down." (Did you know where you were?) "I guess that was the day I thought I was on the ship." When the sister spoke to her, she seemed depressed and said, "If only I had not done those things I might be saved, if I had only gone to church more."

Dec. 3. Seems depressed. She weeps some, says she is sad, "There seems to be something over my heart, so I can't see my little girls." Again: "I should have told you about it first—I should not have bought it"—(refers to buying carbolic acid). She wrote a natural letter but very slowly.

4. There followed then a state lasting for six months, during which the patient was rather inactive, preoccupied, even a little tense at times. Sometimes she did not answer, again at the same interview spoke quite promptly. For the most part the affect was reduced, at other times she appeared a little uneasy, bewildered, or again depressed. She said that sometimes a mist seemed to be over her. Now and then spoke of things looking queer and she asked, when the room was cleaned, "Why do they move things about?" and she added irrelevantly: "I thought the robbers broke into my house and stole my wedding dress and my children's dresses" (refers to the condition during the onset of her psychosis). In the beginning of this state, when asked about the stupor, she spoke again of the "ship" and about going "down, down," but also said that on one occasion she heard beautiful music, was waiting for the last trumpet and was afraid to move. Moreover, she had some ideas referring to the actual situation which were akin to those in the more marked stupor period. Although she admitted she was better, she said on December 8 that she still had queer ideas at times, "I sometimes think the doctor is Uncle Jim" (long dead). She also spoke of other patients looking like dead relatives, and added, "Are

all the spirits that are dead over here?" "We never die here, the spirits are here." But after that date no such ideas recurred, in fact this whole period seems to have been remarkably barren of delusions. Exceptionally isolated ones were noted. Thus, on January 28 it is mentioned that she stated she sometimes felt so lonely, and as though people were against her; and on February 13 she [90] said she felt as though the chair knew what she was talking about. It is also mentioned in January that she wept at times, but this seems not to have been a leading feature at all. In March, when asked why she was not more active and cheerful, her lips began to quiver and she said, "Oh, I thought my children would be cut up in Bellevue." "I don't know why I feel that way about them." She sometimes cried when her friends left her.

5. Then followed a week of a rather faultfinding, self-assertive state, during which she demanded to be allowed to go home, saying indignantly that she was not a wicked woman, had done nothing to be kept a prisoner here; she wanted justice because another patient had called her crazy. But in this period also she said that after the robbery (at home) she felt afraid that her honor would be taken away. When told that her husband had been with her, she said "Yes, but I was afraid they would get into a fight." (You mean you were afraid the other man would kill him?) "No, he is not dead." She further talked of a disagreement she had at that time with her husband, and that she felt then like running away and leading a bad life, but thought of the children. With tears she added: "I would not do anything that is wrong. I have my children to live for." Quite remarkable was the fact that she then told of various erotic experiences in her life, though with a distinctly moral attitude and minimizing them.

6. On *June 16* another state was initiated with peculiar ideas, the setting of which is not known, as she told them only to the nurses. She said that she was not Mrs. W. but the Queen of England, again that she was an actress, or again the wife of a wealthy Mr. B., and that she was going to have a baby. But at night she is said to have been agitated and afraid she was to be executed. She asked to be allowed to go to bed again, then stopped talking, and remained in this mute condition for about a week. She often left her bed and

went back again, remained much with a perplexed expression. On one occasion she put tinsel in her hair saying it was a golden crown.

7. At the end of that time she became freer and more natural, and remained so for three weeks. She occupied herself somewhat. When asked what had happened in the condition preceding, said she thought she was a queen or was to be a queen.

[91] 8. Towards the end of this period she had again three more absorbed days, but when examined on the third of these days got rather talkative and somewhat drifting in her talk on superficial topics.

9. Two days later she began to sing at night, kissed everybody, said it was the anniversary of her meeting her husband, again cried a little, and on the following morning began to sing love songs, with a rather ecstatic mood, and at times stood in an attitude of adoration with her hands raised. This passed over to a more elated state, during which she smiled a good deal, often quite coquettishly; she sang love songs softly; on one occasion put a mosquito netting over her head like a bridal veil; or she held her fingers in the shape of a ring over a flower pinned to her breast. But even during this state she said little, only once spoke of waiting for her wedding ring, and again, when asked why she had been singing, said "I was singing to the man I love." (Why are you so happy?) "Because I am with you" (coquettishly).

This, however, represented the end of the psychosis. She improved rapidly. At first she smiled rather readily, but soon began to occupy herself and made a perfect recovery.

She gave a rather shallow retrospective account about the last phase: at first she said it was natural for people to feel happy at times, and that she did not talk more because the inclination was not there. The only point she added later was that she held her fingers in the shape of a ring because she was thinking of her wedding ring.

She was discharged on *October 11*.

The patient was seen again in *September, 1915*. She then stated that she had been perfectly well until 1912, when she had a breakdown after childbirth. (A childbirth in 1910 had led to no disorder.) The attack lasted six months. She slept poorly, lost weight, and felt weak, depressed, "my strength seemed all gone." In *July, 1915*, following again a childbirth, she was for about six weeks "despondent, weak and tired out."

At the interview she made a very natural, frank impression, and displayed excellent insight.

Case 13. — *Johanna S.* Age: 47. Admitted to the Psychiatric Institute January 23, 1904.

[92] *F. H.* It was claimed that there was no insanity in the family.

P. H. The patient was said to have been bright and rather quick-tempered. She came to the United States from Ireland at the age of 20, worked as a servant, was well liked, and retained her position well.

She was married at 24. After a second confinement, at the age of 26, the patient had her first attack of manic excitement, from which she recovered in four months. She had, subsequently, at the ages of 28, 30, 32, 35, 43, and 45, other attacks of the same nature, each one lasting about four months. No precipitating cause was known for any of them. Only one of the attacks, the fifth, (none were well observed) seems to have shown features different from an elated excitement with irritability. At the end of this attack she was said to have been "dull" for a month.

Her husband died four years before the present admission, evidently soon after her sixth attack.

The present attack:

About two months before admission the patient began, without appreciable cause, to be sleepless, complained of headaches and appeared downhearted and sad. She sat about.

After a week she would not get out of bed and remained in bed until she was sent to the Observation Pavilion, getting up only to go to the closet. She said very little and would not eat much. About a month before admission she began to say that she did not want to live, begged her daughter to throw her out of the window. About two weeks before admission she began to insist that she heard the voice of her brother (living in Ireland) calling her. She got out of bed to look for him.

At the *Observation Pavilion* she was described as slow, looking about in an apprehensive manner, bewildered, dazed, saying "I am dead—there is poison in it (not clear in what)—I am dead, you are dead."

Under Observation: 1. On admission the patient had a coated tongue, foul breath, constipation, lively knee-jerks and a pulse of 110. She appeared dull, inactive, lay in bed with her eyes closed. She would open them when urged but appeared drowsy and her face was strikingly immobile. At times she moaned a little. She could be made to respond in various ways such as [93] shaking her head, or making some motions as though to indicate that she could not give any explanations. All movements were slow. She also responded to a few questions by "I don't know."

Two days after admission the condition was not essentially different except that she was a little uneasy when urged to speak, corrugated her forehead, said "Everything is dark," again "I am very sick," or she turned away her head.

On the fourth day, i.e., January 26, the picture altered, inasmuch as she was much more responsive. She was found sitting up in bed and, at times, a little uneasy. She was slow in her movements and answers, speaking in a whisper and sometimes a little fretfully. The answers, though slow, were, however, by no means given in the shortest possible manner, but with variations, e.g., from "I don't know," to "I could not tell you," or "I can't tell that either." She said herself that everything had "been so dark—it is light now, but it gets so dark sometimes." She denied knowing where she was, even in what city, also denied knowing the month, adding to the latter answer "the nurse can tell you." She could not tell where she had been before coming to the hospital, or how she came. Finally, she also claimed not to know her age, her birthday or the date of her marriage; but she gave the current year correctly, the place where she went to school, the names of some of her teachers, and the year of her arrival in the United States. She also stated in answer to questions that she came to the hospital "to get well." She repeatedly said "I am so sick," or "I am so stupid," or "My mind is mixed up, twisted," or "My mind is not so good," or "I am so tired." What could be obtained of a content was as follows: When she spoke of being "twisted," she said, "I got all kinds of medicine." (How does it affect you?) "Through my head and it made me hot inside." Again, when asked whether anybody had done anything to her, she said "No, I have done wrong myself, by speaking bad of my neighbors." She claimed to hear voices "all over," but could not tell what they said. When, in the evening of that day, the nurse asked her why she did not talk more, she said, "God damn it, I am all twisted, my brain is mixed up, my system is all upset, the doctor made me stupid with questions, and the medicine I have taken made me all stupid and I am inhaling gas now." Then she again settled into a dull state and was found [94] by the physician with immobile expression, slow motions and mute.

2. For about ten days, i.e., from January 27 to February 8, her condition was of a more pronounced character. For the most part she lay in bed with often quite immobile face and with eyes closed, or she looked about in a bewildered manner. She was very inactive, presented a marked resistance in her arms and jaw when passive motions were attempted, or, again, exhibited decided catalepsy. She had to be tube-fed. Once on the 27th of January, when the nurse tried to feed her, she pushed her away and said, "I am dead — I am not home." Sometimes she turned her hands about with slow tremulous movements, looking at them in a bewildered manner.

She usually was mute, except on the few occasions to be mentioned later, as well as on February 3, when she was generally a little more responsive. At that time she could be made to open her eyes, and then replied to a few questions slowly and in a low tone; others were left unanswered. (To the questions where she was and how long she had been here, she replied with "I don't know," but to questions about who the physician and the nurse were, by saying "You are a doctor," and "she is a nurse.")

In the general setting just described there occurred at various times changes in behavior which were as follows: On the evening of the 27th of January she got out of bed and walked about with slow restlessness, saying: "They say I am going to be cut up." On February 1, she was seen for a time making peculiar slow swimming motions with her hands. Again on the 3d of February she got out of bed, walked about slowly, with peculiar steps, as though avoiding stepping on something. Next day (the 4th) she sat up in bed—again made at times her peculiar slow swimming motions. She presented at the same time a peculiar dazed bewildered uneasiness and, when questioned what was the matter, said: "I am—I am—at the bottom of the deep—deep water—oh—oh—the deep—deep—dark water." And when further urged she added with the same manner, "I can't swim—I don't know—but the place"—She did not finish but later again muttered "the deep—deep—dark water." (Do you really think you are in the water?) "I don't know—my head is so bad."

For the following five days this behavior was repeated from time to time, when she would sit up and with bewildered uneasiness make slow swimming motions and mutter when questioned, "I am in the deep, dark water."

Some other emotional responses in reaction to external events must still be mentioned. They were rare. On February 1 the patient's daughter came while she was lying motionless in bed. She slowly extended her hands, tried to speak, and then her eyes filled with tears. Again, at the end of the interview of February 3, after she had made a few replies, she settled down to her usual inactivity and, when further urged to answer, her eyes filled with tears.

3. From about February 9 to February 24 the condition again presented a different aspect, inasmuch as while there was still a marked reduction of activity, she showed this to a decidedly lesser degree. Moreover, there was no bewilderment at any time. No resistance, but cataleptic tendencies were still seen occasionally. There was at no time the peculiar dazed uneasiness and slow restlessness associated with the idea of being in the deep, dark water.

She now dressed herself very slowly, ate slowly but of her own accord, and spoke, though her voice was consistently slow, in a low tone and her words were few.

At the beginning of this period on February 9, when asked how she was, she said "I—I am sick." To the questions as to where she was, how long she had been here and how she had been taken sick, she replied by saying "I don't know." But she knew she was in a hospital, had been here before "many times." (Correct.) She was then again asked for the name of the hospital, but replied "I don't know." So the physician pointed out of the window and asked her what it was that she could see there (the East River). She replied, "It is the dark water. Sometimes I go there and don't come back again—and—something throws me up and I come back." (What has been the matter with you?) "I have been sick all this time." Again, "I can't tell—I am not a good woman—I am very sick." (Why do you say you are not a good woman?) "Oh, I did not do things right."

At a later interview, during the same period, she knew the doctor's name, knew she had seen him at Ward's Island, knew [96] she was in a hospital, but somehow could not connect the present place with Ward's Island. She said she didn't know, when asked where she was, and when questioned about the season, said, after a pause "Summer" (February 15).

We have seen above that she once spoke of not having been a good woman. She repeated this on February 10, said "I have done lots of harm, I have been a bad woman all my life." Again: "I had bad thoughts." (What kind?) "I have forgotten all about them." It should be added that at this interview she also said, "My mind is better now."

On February 25 there was a sudden change. She laughed when a funny remark was made on the ward. Later, when the physician came to her, she still lay in bed inactive and had to be urged considerably at first, but presently began to laugh good-naturedly and quite freely commented on the funny remark she had heard earlier in the morning, and on peculiarities of some patients. She spoke quite freely and without constraint. But it was striking how little account of the condition she had gone through could be obtained from her. She either turned the questions off by flippant remarks, or said she did not know. The only information obtained was that she had been sick since Christmas, felt like a dummy, that she had lost track of time, and did not know how she had felt during that period. When asked why she had not spoken, she said, "I couldn't, I had a jumping toothache," or she said, "Ask the nurse, she put it down in the book." Or again she said, "Did you ever get drunk? That is the way I felt. I felt like dead."

She soon developed a lobar pneumonia and died.

The following typical case of partial stupor is quoted as an example of delusions appearing only during the onset.

Case 14.—*Maggie H.* Age: 26. Admitted to the Psychiatric Institute February 8, 1905.

F. H. The father died when 33. The mother was living. Psychopathic tendencies were denied.

P. H. The husband and brother stated that the patient was [97] natural, capable, rather jolly. She married about a year before admission and shortly became pregnant. During the pregnancy she was rather nervous and had various forebodings, among which were that the child might be born deformed, or that she would die in childbirth.

The baby was born three weeks before admission. The patient seemed much worried immediately after the childbirth, fretted about not having enough milk, was quite concerned about her husband and did not want him to leave her side. The brother stated that about this time the patient heard that the husband was out of work. She worried about this and told her sister so. She also began to say that her head was getting queer. On the fifth day after childbirth, a change came over the patient. She cried and said she was going to die. She also spoke of poison in the food and accused the husband of unfaithfulness. The next day she became silent, "did not seem to want to have anything to do with anybody," lay in bed, had a tendency to pull the covers over her head and scarcely ever spoke. But during this period she continued to look after the baby faithfully. Sometimes she clung to her husband, saying she was afraid he was going to die.

After recovery the patient said that while she was at home she thought she saw bodies lying about.

At the *Observation Pavilion* she was quiet and apathetic, indifferent to environment and could not be induced to speak. She soiled, refused food, and was resistive when anything was done to her.

Under Observation: 1. On admission the patient was fairly well nourished but looked rather anemic and weak. The temperature was normal, the pulse a little irregular but of normal frequency, the tongue coated. She lay inactive but looked about, and the facial expression sometimes changed as she did this. Any interference met with intense resistance. There was no catalepsy. In contradistinction to this inactivity and resistance, natural, free motions were observed at times, as, for example, when she arranged her pillows. She did not speak and could not be made to answer.

For the rest of the first week she made no attempt to speak, except once when she seemed to attempt to return a "good morn [98] ing," or on another occasion, when the nurse tried to feed her, she said, in quite a natural tone, "I can feed myself." The resistance to interference remained in a variable degree, and was at times quite strong. It was largely passive, though not infrequently associated with a scowl, or she moved away when approached. She sometimes looked dull and stared, again she looked determined, "disdainful," or scowled; or she looked about watching others, sometimes only out of the corners of her eyes. She had to be spoon-fed at times, again she ate naturally when the food was brought. Repeatedly, when taken out of bed, though she resisted at first, she dressed with natural free motions. She always retracted promptly from pin pricks.

Towards the end of the week she even complied at times with a request to do some work, but on the same day she would remain passive, with a look of disdain, or resist intensely when interfered with, e.g., when an attempt was made to make her sit down. She never soiled and never showed any catalepsy.

2. Then the condition changed, inasmuch as the marked resistance ceased entirely, and the mutism gave way first to slow and low answers, and later to much freer speech, though the inactivity improved only gradually. Thus at the examination on February 19, though she was quite inactive, she answered some questions, albeit in whispers and briefly. This was the case when questioned about the year, month and date, which she gave correctly, but she merely shook her head when asked how long she had been here, why she was here, what was the matter with her. Once she smiled appropriately. Later she became freer in speech, with a more natural tone, although her answers continued to be short. Not infrequently, when asked to calculate or to write, she would not coöperate, saying "This has nothing to do with my getting well," or (later) "What has that

got to do with my going home?" or she would simply say she did not want to. Improvement in her listlessness and inactivity was more gradual.

The prevailing affective state was indefinite. She denied repeatedly that she was depressed, though later she admitted once being downhearted, yet it seems that even then her mood was not so much one of sadness as of a slight resentment. On one occasion, however, she showed some tears when asked about the baby. She repeatedly expressed the wish to go home, but not in a pleading, rather in a resentful, way, saying she would never be better here, that the questions which were asked had nothing to do with her going home, that she would be all right if she went home. She never admitted that she had ever been sick enough to be taken to a hospital, though she quite appreciated that there had been something the matter with her head at home and in the hospital. She stated, in answer to questions, that she had a peculiar feeling in the head which she could not explain, that she could not remember so well as formerly. Once she said, "I hear so much around here that my head gets so full."

When towards the end she was questioned about her condition, i.e., the reason for her resistance, her mutism, and her refusal of food, she said that then she "wanted to be left alone"; that she did not eat "because she did not want food," and she also spoke of not having had any interest.

She was discharged on April 29, i.e., about ten weeks after admission before she had become entirely free.

The last case is interesting in that a depressive onset to a deep stupor was observed in the Institute. It was characterized by constant repetitions of a request to be killed.

Case 15.—*Meta S.* Age: 16. Admitted to the Psychiatric Institute June 26, 1902.

F. H. The father was dead, and the mother living abroad. Not much could be learned about them and the immediate family.

P. H. An aunt who gave the anamnesis had known the patient only since she came to the United States, a year before admission. After her arrival the patient at once went to work as a servant. It was claimed that her employer liked her, but that she was rather slow about the work. The only trouble known was that she sometimes complained of indigestion. She went to see her aunt about once every two weeks.

Three weeks before admission, when the patient visited her aunt, she seemed quieter than usual. Further, she spoke about sending money home on the *Kaiser Wilhelm der Grosse*, which was thought peculiar because she had no money, and on a walk [100] through a cemetery said "I would like to be here too." At the time this did not impress the aunt as very peculiar. The patient continued to work until nine days before admission. The employer then sent for the aunt and said the patient had been very quiet for about two weeks, and that she now had become more abnormal. She suddenly had begun to cry, said the police had come, claimed, without foundation, that she had "stolen," and kept repeating "I have done it, I will not do it again." The aunt took her home with her. There she was quite dejected, cried, spoke of killing herself (wanted to jump out of the window, wanted to get a knife). On the whole, she said very little, but when the aunt pressed her to say why she was so worried, she said she had allowed men to kiss her and had taken money from them. It is claimed that she never menstruated.

After recovery the patient herself described the onset as follows: Ever since she came to this country she had been homesick, and felt especially lonesome for some months before admission. She knew, however, of no precipitating cause, in spite of what she had said to the aunt and what she said at first under observation. She consistently denied that anything had happened with young men. A short time before she left her place (she left it nine days before admission) she could not work, began to accuse herself of being a bad girl and of having stolen. Then she was taken to the aunt's house. There she wanted to die.

Under Observation: 1. On admission the patient appeared depressed, sat with downcast expression, looking up rarely. She spoke in a low tone and slowly. But, in spite of delay, she answered all questions, knew where she was and gave an account of the place where she had worked. When questioned about trouble with men, she claimed that a man who lived in the same house where she worked had tried to make her "lie on the bed," but that she refused; that later a man had assaulted her and had after that repeatedly come to her room when she was alone. Yet when asked whether she worried about this, she denied it.

2. For eight days her condition was sometimes one of marked reduction of activity, with preoccupation. She sat in a dejected attitude, and had to be urged to do anything. Sometimes she was very slow in greeting and slow in answering, and said very little. But whenever spoken to she was apt to cry and this might lead to such distress that the reduction of activity was no longer to be seen. Thus on June 28, when greeted, she began to cry and say, "Oh, what have I done!—Oh, just cut my head off—Oh, please what have I done—I have given my hand." (Tell me the whole story.) Imploringly and with hands clasped: "No, I can't do it—just cut my head off, please, please." (Why can you not tell me?) "Oh, what have I done!" The imploring to cut her head off was then several times repeated, and she could not be made to answer orientation questions. On June 29 she became agitated spontaneously and cried loudly, saying, "Oh, let me go home and die with my father." She was then put to bed, and when seen she could not be made to answer orientation questions. But when asked whether she had seen the physician before, she said, "I saw you yesterday." She could not be made, however, to say how long she had been here, "I think a"—not finishing the sentence. Although she would not answer further, she presently began to say "Oh, cut my head off—oh, where is my papa and mamma?" When told that her people were in Germany and that she could go back to them, she said "I haven't any money to pay it." Then she wanted to know if she was to pay for her board and bed and said she could not do it.

Again, on July 1, although she had been quite preoccupied, inactive and silent, she began to say when greeted, "Oh, please cut my head off." But she then answered some questions, said she had not worked enough. On questioning, she explained it was not that the work had been too much, but that she had been nervous, had tried to work as much as the servant next door, but could do only half as much, "Oh, I ought to have worked."

Repeatedly on other occasions she begged, with distress, to have her head cut off or to be killed. Frequently there were statements of self-blame: she ought to have worked more, was lazy or "I am not worthy"; or she said she had lied and stolen; or again, "I have not paid for these beds and I cannot," or "I am a bad girl."

3. For a month she presented a more marked reduction of activity. She sat about with a dejected look, often gazed in a preoccupied manner, or she stood or walked around slowly. Sometimes she had to be spoon-fed. At other times she ate slowly. Toward the latter part of this period, a distinct tendency to [102] catalepsy appeared. During this period, too, as a rule (though not always), she would cry when spoken to. A few times she would make some ineffectual motions when questioned, but she scarcely ever spoke.

4. Then followed a period again lasting about one month in which the picture was at times one of still greater inactivity. She would retain uncomfortable positions, allow flies to crawl over her face. She presented resistance in the jaws, did not react to pin pricks. She sometimes sat with eyes closed or, with an immobile face, the eyes stared with little blinking. The catalepsy was more decided. She often would not swallow solid food but swallowed fluid. Again she held her saliva, sometimes drooled. Once she held her urine and had to be catheterized. When spoken to she once smiled at a joke, sometimes there was no response, but as a rule there were tears or flushing of the face. On the physical side, there were marked dermatographia and, for a time, towards the end of the period, profuse sweating. Throughout the stupor proper her temperature was between 99° and 100° as a rule.

5. The period which followed and which lasted about two months was characterized, like the one just described, by marked stupor symptoms, associated, however, with more resistance, while the crying practically disappeared. On the other hand, a number of plainly angry reactions were seen and, towards the end, smiling and laughing. She lay in bed, on her back, staring, allowing the flies to crawl over her face; retained uncomfortable positions without correcting them, and her arms often showed a decided tendency to catalepsy. Sometimes she soiled. She constantly held saliva in her mouth, though she did not often drool. She was totally mute, did

not respond in any way except in the manner to be presently indicated. She had to be tube-fed a good part of the time, was quite resistive when an attempt was made to open her mouth. When attended to by the nurse, she was apt to make herself stiff. But as a rule, she was not resistive to passive motions when tested. On a few occasions she had, as was stated, marked angry outbursts. Thus on one occasion when her temperature was taken she angrily pushed the nurse away and then struggled vigorously. On another occasion, when the bed-pan was put under her, she threw it away angrily and struck [103] the nurse; once she did the same with the feeding tube. She struck a patient, on another occasion, when the latter came to her bed. On two occasions she suddenly threw herself headlong on the floor. Towards the end of the period, when the blood-pressure was taken, she smiled and then laughed out loud. She could be made to smile again later.

6. The last period, before the more definite improvement, lasted about a month. She was inactive and slow, ate slowly (feeding no longer necessary), and was mute. But she did not stare, was no longer resistive, no longer held saliva. She appeared indifferent, but could be made to smile quite readily when spoken to. On one occasion she laughed out loud when a comical toy was shown her, again was amused at a party. In the beginning of the period she was once seen to cry a little when sitting by herself, and at the same time wept a little when spoken to, but this was now isolated. Towards the end of the period she spoke a little, asked for paper and pencil and wrote: "Dear Mother. — I only take up the pencil in order to write you a few lines. We are all cheerful and in good health and hope that you are the same and we congratulate you on your birthday 19th of December that I have not written to you for a long time were in the same ..." (Translated.) This was written very slowly.

On the day after this letter she was distinctly freer, talked a little to the nurse and then improved rapidly. A week after this, January 16, she is described as quite free in her talk and activity, but when asked about the psychosis she merely shrugged her shoulders. However, mere extensive retrospective accounts were taken later.

The retrospective accounts were obtained on January 24 and March 13. As these two accounts do not seem to be fundamentally different for the period of the psychosis, they may here for the sake of brevity be combined.

She remembered clearly going to the Observation Pavilion, and feeling frightened, as she did not know where she was going and what they were going to do with her. She knew when she was in the Observation Pavilion and had a good recollection of the place, also of the transfer to the hospital, the ward she came to, who spoke to her, etc. She did not know what the place was until the doctor told her a day or two after admission. Unfor [104] tunately definite incidents were inquired into only for the first part (July). But she remembered those clearly. She also claimed to remember all visits which were made to her by her friends, but it was not specifically determined whether there was a period of less clear recollection or not. However, she remembered the tube-feeding, which occurred only during the more marked stupor. Her desire to be killed, to have her head cut off, she recalled but claimed not to know why she wanted to be killed. However, she remembered worrying about being bad, about the fact that she could not "pay for the beds," etc.

Her mutism and refusal of food she was unable to account for. She could not talk, her "tongue would not move." As regards ideas during the more stuporous period, she claimed that (when quite inactive) she heard voices but did not recall what they said. But she remembered having dreams at that time "of fire," "of her dead father and of home."

In a survey of thirty-six consecutive cases of definite stupor, literal death ideas were found in all but one case. They seem to be commonest during the period immediately preceding the stupor, as all but five of these cases spoke of death while the psychosis was incubating. From this we may deduce that the stupor reaction is consequent on ideas of death, or, to put it more guardedly, that death ideas and stupor are consecutive phenomena in the same fundamental process. Two-thirds of these patients interrupted the stupor symptoms to speak of death or attempt suicide, which would lead us to suppose that this intimate relationship still continued. One-quarter gave a retrospective account of delusions of being dead, being in Heaven, and so on. From this we may suspect that in many cases there may be a thought content, although the patient's mind may [105] seem to be a complete blank. It is important to note that when a retrospective account is gained, the delusions are practically always of death or something akin to it, such as being in prison, feeling paralyzed, stiff, and so on.

In the one case of the thirty-six who presented no literal death ideas, the psychosis was characterized essentially by apathy and mild confusion, a larval stupor reaction. It began with a fear of fire, smelling smoke and a conviction that her house would burn down. It is surely not straining interpretation to suggest that this phobia was analogous to a death fear. When one considers the incompleteness of anamneses not taken *ad hoc* (for these are largely old cases) and that the rule in stupor is silence, the consistence with which this content appears is striking.

To exemplify the form in which these delusional thoughts occur we may cite the following: Henrietta H. (Case 8) said, retrospectively, that she thought she was dead, that she saw shadows of dead friends laid out for burial, that she saw scenes from Heaven and earth. Annie K. (Case 5) claimed to have had the belief that she was going to die, and to have had visions of her dead father and dead aunt, who were calling her. She also thought that all the family were dead and that she was in a cemetery. Rosie K. (Case 11) said she had the idea that she wanted to die and that she refused food for that purpose, and during the stupor she sometimes held her breath until she was cyanotic. Mary F. (Case [106] 3), before her stupor became profound, spoke of the hereafter, of being in Calvary and in Heaven. In this case, as well as in the above-mentioned Henrietta H., we find, therefore, associated with "death" the closely related idea of Heaven. Whether Calvary merely referred to the cemetery (Mt. Calvary Cemetery) or leads over to the motif of crucifixion, cannot be decided. It is, however, clear that this latter motif may be associated with that of death, as is shown in Charlotte W. (Case 12), who, during intervals when the inactivity lifted, spoke of having been dead, of spirits having told her that she must die, of having gone to Heaven, of God having told her that she must die on the cross like Christ. But this patient also showed in a second subperiod of her stupor another content. She said: "It was like water. I was going down." Or again, she spoke of having gone "under the ground"; "I went down, down in a coffin." She spoke of having gone down "into a dark hole," "down, down, up, up"; again, of having been "on a ship." We shall see in the further course of our study that this type of content occurs not at all infrequently.

The internal relationship among the different ideas associated with stupor: Before we go any further it may be advisable to examine the meaning of such ideas when they arise in other settings than those of the psychoses. If we consider these ideas of death, Heaven, of going under ground, being in water, in a boat, etc., we are impressed with the similarity which they bear to certain mythological [107] motifs. This is, of course, not the place to enter into this topic more than briefly. We are here concerned with a clinical study, and therefore, among other tasks, with the interrelationship of symptoms, but for that purpose it is necessary to point out how these ideas seen in stupor can be shown to have, not only a connection amongst each other, when viewed as deep-seated human strivings, but also are closely related to, or identical with, ideas found in mythology.

To one's conscious mind death may be not only the dreaded enemy who ends life, but also the friend who brings relief from all conflict, strife and effort. Death may, therefore, well express a shrinking from adaptation and reality, and as such may symbolize one of the most deep-seated yearnings of the human soul. But from time immemorial man has associated with this yearning another one, one which, without the adaptation to reality being made, yet includes a certain attempt at objectivation, the desire for rebirth. We need not enter further into possible symbols for death *per se*, but it is quite necessary to speak briefly of the symbolic forms in which the striving for rebirth has ever found expression. The reader will find a large material collected in various writings on mythology, for the psychological interpretation of which reference may be made to Jung's "Wandlungen und Symbole der Libido" and Rank's "Mythos von der Geburt des Helden." From them it appears how old are the symbols for rebirth, and how they deal chiefly with [108] water and earth, and the idea of being surrounded by and enclosed in a small space. Thus we find a sinking into the water of the sea, enclosure in something which swims on or in the water, such as a casket, or a basket, or a fish, or a boat; again, we find descent into the earth. The striving for rebirth might be assumed to have adopted these expressions or symbols on account of the concrete way in which the human mind knows birth to take place. The tendency for concrete expression of abstract notions causes the desire for another existence to appear, first as a rebirth fantasy and then as a return to the mother's body. One thinks of Job's cry, "Naked came I from my mother's womb and naked shall I return thither," as an example of the literal comparison of death with birth. We need only refer to the myths of Moses and the older one of Osiris, and the many myths of the birth of the hero, to call to the mind of the reader the examples which mythology furnishes. There is probably not one of the ideas expressed by these patients which cannot be duplicated in myths. We have, therefore, a right to speak of these ideas as "primitive," and to see in them, not only deep-seated strivings of the human soul, but to recognize in them an essential inner relationship. It is especially this last fact to which at this point we wish to call attention: that without any obvious connection the fantasies of our forefathers recur in the delusions of our stupor cases. We presume that in each case they represent a fulfillment of a primitive human demand. In one of our cases a vision of [109] Heaven and a conscious longing to be there was followed by a stupor. On recovery the patient compared her condition to that of a butterfly just hatched from a cocoon. No clearer simile of mental rebirth could be given.

Brief survey of the ideas associated with the states preceding the stupor: If we now return to the study of the further occurrence of such ideas in the cases described, we find motifs, similar to those seen in the stupor, in the period which immediately precedes the more definite stupor reaction. Indeed we find the ideas there with greater regularity. In Meta S. (Case 15) the stupor followed upon six days with reduced activity and crying, with self-accusation, but also with entreaties to be allowed to go home and die with her father. At the very onset of her breakdown, the desire for death had also occurred. Anna G. (Case 1) expressed a wish to be with her dead father, and, at the visit of a cousin, she had a vision of the latter's dead mother. A second attack of this same patient began with the idea that the dead father was calling her. Maggie H. (Case 14) saw dead bodies, and during outbursts of greater anxiousness, she thought her husband was going to die. In Caroline De S. (Case 2) the psychosis began with a coarse excitement, with statements about being killed, with entreaties to be shot, with the idea of going to Heaven, again with frequent calling out that she loved her father (who was dead since her ninth year), while immediately before the stupor the condition passed into a muttering state [110] in which she spoke of being killed. Mary D. (Case 4) began by worrying over the father's death (dead four years before), had visions of the latter beckoning, and she heard voices saying, "You will be dead." Mary F. (Case 3) had a vision of "a person in white," and thought she was going to die. In Henrietta H. (Case 8) the stupor was preceded by nine days of elation, with ideas of shooting and of war, but this had commenced with hearing voices of dead friends, and with ideas that somebody wanted to kill her family. In the case of Annie K. (Case 5) we find before the stupor a state of worry, with reduction of activity, and then a vision of the dead father coming for her. In Charlotte W. (Case 12) the stupor was preceded by a state of preoccupation, with distress and entreaties to be saved, partly from being put into a big hole, partly from the electric chair.

We see, therefore, in the introductory phase of the stupor in almost every case ideas of death, and in one case an idea belonging to the rebirth motif, namely, of being put into a dark hole. In well-observed cases apparently we do not find the stupor reaction without either coincident or preceding ideas of death.

Relation of death and rebirth ideas with affect: In order to investigate the relation of these ideas to the affective condition associated with them, it will be necessary to study not only the abstract ideational content but the special formulation in which the content appears. In looking over the enumera [111] tion of the ideas given above, it is very clear that these formulations differed considerably from each other. A priori we would say that it is, psychologically, a very different matter whether a person expresses a desire to die, or has the idea that he will die or is dead, or says he will be killed. We associate the first with sadness, the last with fear, while our daily experience does not give us so much information about the delusion of being dead. A vivid expectation of death is usually accompanied by either fear or resignation.

In studying the ideas which we obtained from the patients by retrospective account after the psychosis or from a retrospective account during freer intervals, it is, of course, difficult, especially in the former case, to say whether they have persisted for any length of time. Probably in most instances this was not the case, and we must remember in this connection that in a considerable number of cases the patients recalled no ideas whatever.

Of the five cases which we may consider as types, Henrietta H. (Case 8) and Mary F. (Case 3) formulated their ideas simply as *accepted facts* during the stupor. The former thought she was dead, saw dead friends laid out for burial, and scenes from Heaven and earth. The latter spoke, during the stupor, of being in "Calvary," "the hereafter," or "Heaven." We have seen that these stupors were essentially affectless reactions and we can therefore say that, so far as these two cases are concerned, the ideas thus formulated were not associated with any affect.

[112] Annie K. (Case 5) was a little different. During the stupor she made a few utterances about priests and "all being dead," and retrospectively she said that she had thought she was in the cemetery, was going to die, that she had repeated visions of her dead father and once of a dead aunt calling her; that she had thought her family were dead, again that the baby (who was born just before the psychosis) was dead. The formulation is therefore less one of fact than of something prospective, something which is coming—the *going* to die. Correlated, perhaps, with this anticipation were slight modifications of the usual apathy. The patient often had an expression of bewilderment. She was also more in contact with her environment than many stuporous patients are, for, not infrequently, she would look at what was going on about her. Her apathy was also broken into in a marked degree by her active resistiveness, which was sometimes accompanied by plain anger. It seems that a prospect of death may occur in other instances in a totally affectless state. We have recently seen it in a partial stupor during which the patient spoke and had this persistent idea in a setting of complete apathy. We see here also, as in one of the former cases, the idea of other members of the family being dead.

More difficult and deserving more discussion are the two remaining cases, Rosie K. (Case 11) and Charlotte W. (Case 12). Rosie K. showed a peculiar condition. She said, retrospectively, that during the stupor she had the desire to die and that for this [113] purpose she refused food. Moreover, she was repeatedly seen to hold her breath with great insistence, though without affect. This is worth noting. We are in the habit in psychiatry to say in a case like this that "there is no affect," and yet there is evidently a considerable "push" behind the action. We shall later have to mention in detail a patient whom we regard as belonging in the group of stupor reactions, and who for a time made insistent, impulsive and most determined suicidal attempts, yet with a peculiar blank affectless facial expression and with shouting which was more like that of a huckster than one in despair. Here also, then, there was a great deal of "push," yet not associated with that which we call in psychiatry an affect. In both instances we see acts which we are in the habit of calling for this very reason "impulsive." Evidently this is an important psychological problem which leads directly into the psychology of affects and deserves further study. For the present it is enough to say that with a different formulation—that of wishing to die—there is here not, as in other psychoses, a definite affect, such as sadness or despair, but no affect, though there may be a good deal of "push" or impulsiveness.

The case of Charlotte W. (Case 12) is a complicated one, for she had short stupor periods with inactivity, catalepsy, resistiveness, etc., which were interrupted with freer spells. A careful analysis of her history has been instructive and justifies a detailed and lengthy discussion. For the purpose in [114] hand it is necessary to separate the ideas which she expressed only in the freer periods (during which some affect was at times seen) into those which referred retrospectively to the stupor phase and those which referred to the freer periods themselves.

We find that the time during which more marked stupor symptoms appeared may be divided into two subperiods. This is not possible in regard to the manifestations belonging to the general reaction, which seem to have undergone no decided change, but only in regard to the form of the delusions. In this we find there was a first phase in which ideas of death and Heaven (and crucifixion) occurred, and a second phase in which ideas were present which belonged essentially to the motif of rebirth but which were also associated with ideas of Heaven.

About the first subperiod she said: "I was mesmerized," or "I thought I was dead," or "God told me I must die on the cross as He did," or "I went to Heaven in spirit." About the second subperiod she said retrospectively: "We were on a ship and we were 'most drowned.'" "It was like water, I was going down, down." She said she saw the people of the hospital and "it was all full of water"; or again, "I went under the ground and it was full of water and every one got drowned and a sharp thing struck me"; or "I was out on a ship and I went down in a coffin." She claimed she put up her arms to save the ship. Again she spoke of having gone into a dark hole. She also said: "One day I was in a coffin—that was the day I went to Heaven." [115] "They used to be coming up and down, that was the day I was coming up in a ship or going down." And when shown her picture in a cataleptic attitude, she said: "That must have been when I went to Heaven—everything seemed strange, things seemed to go up and down—I guess that was the day I thought I was on the ship." Finally she also said: "Once I heard beautiful music—I was waiting for the last trumpet—I was afraid to move."

We see, therefore, that most of the ideas which she thus spoke of retrospectively as having been in her mind during this stupor, and which belonged both to the death and the rebirth motifs were formulated as facts (as in the cases of Henrietta H. and Mary F. above mentioned). It was, moreover, a condition which was accepted without protest. Here again an affect was not associated with these ideas, and when the patient was asked whether she had not been frightened, she said herself, "No, I just lay there." The idea that God told her she would have to die on the cross like Christ, is, in the religious form, like the beckoning of the father with Henrietta H. The only exception to the claim that the ideas were formulated as facts and accepted as inevitable seems to be the statement that she held up her arms to save the ship. This would seem to be, in contradistinction to the rest, a formulation as a more dangerous situation. However, this was isolated and we can do no more than to determine main tendencies. We must expect, especially in such variable conditions as we see in this patient, to find occasional inconsistencies.

[116] In summing up we may say, therefore, that so far as the stupor itself is concerned, the ideas are formulated as a rule:—

1. As accepted facts (being dead, being in a ship, etc.).
2. As accepted prospects (going to die).
3. As the wish to die.

In the first two types the ideas are not associated with affect; in the third, though not associated with affect, they are combined with "impulsive" suicidal attempts.

In order not to tear apart the analysis of Charlotte W. (Case 12) too much, we may begin our study of the intervals and the conditions preceding the stupors with the ideas which this patient produced when the stupor lifted somewhat. We shall see that the ideas are closely related to those mentioned above but formulated differently.

It will be remembered that Charlotte W. had freer intervals when she responded and was less constrained generally, and that it was in these that the ideas above mentioned were gathered. Since they were spoken of in the past tense, we regarded them as not belonging to the actual situation but to the more stuporous period. It seems tempting now to see whether the ideas which are expressed in the present tense are different in character, the general aim being to discover whether any tendencies can be found in regard to the types and formulations of delusions associated with different clinical pictures. We see [117] that on November 2 the patient, when speaking much more freely than before, said she had felt that she was mesmerized, was dead, and that she had gone to Heaven, ideas which we have taken up above as belonging to the stupor period. In addition to speaking much more freely in these intervals, she showed at times some affect. Thus to the physician whom she called Christ, she said, with tears, "You came to tell me what was right," or again with tears, "I will have to be crucified," or she spoke in a depressed manner about her children, "I can't see them any more," "I must stay here till I die," and she spoke of having to stay here till she picked her eyes and her brains out; or she claimed her husband or her children had to pick them out. Once she exclaimed crossly and with tears, "You are trying to keep me from Jim" (husband). Another idea was not plainly associated with affect. She said she had come back from Heaven, "The wedding ring kept me on Earth." What strikes one about these formulations is that they are, on the one hand, sometimes associated with an affect, and that, on the other hand, they refer much more to her actual life, her marriage, her husband, her children. At least this seems to be a definite tendency. A similar tendency may be seen later: On November 4, while generally stuporous, this suddenly lifted for a short time, and with feeble voice she uttered some depressive ideas. She said she wanted to go to a convent, that it would be better if she were dead, that she [118] could not do anything right. On November 5 and 6 she said she wanted to go to Jim in Heaven (in contradistinction to the retrospective statements that she had gone to Heaven), and on the 8th, when she had the idea of being in a boat, she said with some anger that she had wanted to get her husband into the boat, but that the doctor kept him out and took his place.

Later there were at times ideas expressed which referred to the actual situation or essentially depressive ideas in a depressive setting. Thus on December 3 she appeared sad, retarded, and spoke of not being able to see her children and that she had done wrong in buying carbolic acid (her suicidal attempt). So far as this case is concerned, therefore, we do find a distinct tendency for the ideas which refer to the more stuporous condition to differ from those which refer to the actual situation in the freer intervals, a difference which we may formulate by saying that, though primitive ideas are expressed, the tendency seems to be to connect them more with actual life, or that the primitive character is lost and the ideas take on a more depressive character with a depressive affect. A few words should be added in regard to the peculiar ideas that she or her husband or her child had to pick out her eyes (or her brain). It is probable that this idea belongs to the motif of sacrifice (the *Opfer motiv* of Jung) into which we need not enter further, except to say that in this instance it was plainly connected, like [119] some of the other ideas just spoken of, with the real situation of her life (husband, children).

It will now be necessary to examine the earlier state of Charlotte W. The condition preceding the stupor set in with pre-occupation, slow talk and slight distress. During the time she asked to be given one more chance, she said to the husband she would not see him again. Then followed a day when she was very slow and with moaning said she was going to be put into a dark hole. Again on the next, when speaking more freely, she begged to be saved from the electric chair, and also said, "Don't kill me, make me true to my husband," etc. [Again the connection with real life!] We see here the idea of death and especially an idea pertaining to the rebirth motif in a setting of distress and slowness, as an introduction to the stupor which had in it both of these motifs. We must leave it undecided whether it is accidental or not that the distress was associated with more slowness (i.e., more marked stupor traits) when she spoke of the dark hole than when she spoke of the electric chair or death. But what interests us is that distress and reduction of activity (not sadness and reduction of activity, which seems as a rule to have a different content) are here associated with ideas seen in stupor but formulated as prospective dangers. We know from experience that we often find associated with the fear of dying considerable freedom of action, and we see at times in involution states conditions with freedom of motion and marked anxiety, whereas the [120] ideas seem to belong to the motif of rebirth; e.g., the fear of being boiled in a tank. [A]

In this connection, however, two other cases should be taken up which show a condition which reminds one somewhat of that we have just discussed, but in which the rebirth motif appeared, not as prospective, but, as in the stupor, as an actual situation. At the same time this situation was not passively accepted but conceived as a dangerous situation. The significant phenomenon in both these conditions was that there was not anxiety with freedom of action but a bewildered uneasiness with marked reduction of activity.

The first case is that of Johanna S., whose history has been given in this chapter. It will be observed that in the fourth period the patient presented two days of typical stupor with the idea that she was dead. We are familiar with this. But this was followed by several days of bewildered uneasiness and slow restlessness, with ideas that she was at the bottom of the deep, dark water and for a time she made attempts at stepping out of the water or swimming motions. All of this was in a general setting of reduction of activity with bewildered uneasiness. In the ideas about being at the bottom of the deep, dark water, we recognize again the re [121] birth motif, yet the situation is not accepted but attempts are made by the patient to save herself, i.e., the attitude is one in which the situation is taken to be one of danger. It is interesting in this connection that immediately following this state there was one day of ordinary retardation with sadness and ideas of being bad and sick. That is, when the element of anxiety, the uneasiness, disappeared and sadness supervened, the rebirth ideas were no longer present.

In Mary C. (See Chapter II, Case 7) we have, unfortunately, not a direct observation, but we have, at any rate, a description from the Observation Pavilion which seems so plain that we should be justified in using it here. The condition we refer to is described as a dazed uneasiness, with ideas of being shut up in a ship, of the ship being closed up so that no one could get out, of the boat having gone down, of the people turning up. We should add here that the condition was not followed by a typical stupor. Essentially it was a retardation, in which only on one occasion was a definite akinesis observed. During this phase she soiled her bed. Perhaps the persistent complaint of inability to take in the environment belonged also more to the retardation of stupor than to that of depression. We have again, therefore, in this initial phase, a similar situation, namely, ideas belonging essentially to the rebirth motif, formulated as of a threatening character if not as actually dangerous.

We can say, therefore, that what characterizes [122] these three cases, and brings them together, is the fact that all three had ideas belonging to the rebirth motif, but formulated as dangerous situations. Associated with this there was not a typical anxiety with the relative freedom of activity belonging to this state, but an anxiety or distress or uneasiness with traits of stupor reaction, namely, slow movements, lack of contact with the environment, and a dazed facial expression. It would seem that these facts could scarcely be accidental but that they must have a deeper significance. As a discussion of this belongs, however, more into the psychological part of this study, we shall defer it for the present, and be satisfied with pointing out here the clinical facts of observation.

In brief, then, our findings as to the ideational content of the benign stupor are as follows: From the utterances during the incubation period of the psychosis, from the ideas expressed in interruptions of the deep stupor, as well as from the memories of recovered patients, we find an extraordinary paucity and uniformity of autistic thoughts. They are concerned with death, often as a plain delusion of being no longer alive, or with the closely related fancy of rebirth. The rule is a setting of apathy for these ideas, but when they are formulated so as to connect them with the real life and problems of the patient, or when rebirth is represented as a dangerous situation, some affect, usually one of distress, may appear.

Footnotes:

[6] Kirby, *loc. cit.*, pointed out that stupor showed resemblance to feigned death in animals, that the reaction suggested a shrinking from life and that ideas of death were common.

[A] We may mention that since this study was made we risked a prediction of stupor, which events justified, in the case of a patient who showed expectation of death without affect. Such opportunities are rare, however, since we usually do not see these cases till the stupor symptoms are manifest. It would be unsafe to dogmatize on the basis of such meager material.

[123]

CHAPTER VI
AFFECT

The most constant and significant symptom in the stupor reaction is the change in affect. This extends from mere quietness in the mildest phases of the disease through the stage of indifference where apathy replaces the normal reactions of the personality, to the final condition of complete inactivity in the vegetative stupor where all mental life seems to have ceased. It seems as though there were, as a pathognomonic sign of the morbid process, a lack of energy and loss of the normal *élan vital*.

We may say, in fact, that the establishment of a specific type of emotional change is justification for classifying all milder stupor reactions with the deep stupors. In other words, our reason for the enlargement of the stupor group to include all apathetic reactions (except those of dementia præcox) is the belief that this dulling of the emotional response is as specific a type of emotional change as is anxiety, depression or elation. Perhaps it would be more accurate to say that this clinical group is founded on the symptom complex which is built around apathy. There is never any resemblance between apathy and the mood of elation or anxiety. [124] A discrimination from depression is the only differentiation worth discussion.

The first point that should be made is that there is a difference between marked depression and the mood of stupor. In the former we get a retardation with a feeling of blocking, rather than of an absence of energy. The expression of the patient is one of dejection, not of vacancy, which bespeaks a mood of sadness, even when the patient is so retarded as to be mute and therefore incapable of describing his emotions. Running through all the stages of stupor, however, there is an emptiness, an indifference that is in striking contrast to the positive pain that is felt or expressed by the depressed patient. It may be objected, of course, that this apathy really represents the final stage in the emotional blocking of the depressed individual, but the development of stupor and recovery from it shows an entirely different type of process. A deep depression recovers by changing the point of view from a feeling of unworthiness and self-blame to one of normality. The stuporous case, on the other hand, evidences merely less and less indifference, and more and more interest in his environment and in himself as he gets well.

The associated symptoms are no less dissimilar. The difficulty in thinking which troubles the depressed patient is slight in proportion to his emotional gloom, and he feels himself to be much more incompetent intellectually than examination proves him to be. On the other hand, in the stupor reac [125] tion we find that the thinking disorder runs hand in hand with the apathy and that the intellectual capacity of the patient is really markedly interfered with, as can be shown by more or less objective tests. A mere slowing of thought processes accompanied by subjective feeling of effort is the limit reached in true depression, while it is merely the beginning of the intellectual disorder in stupor, for one meets with retardation symptoms only in the partial stupors. The slowing in these cases seems to represent an early stage of the intellectual disturbance which reaches its acme in the mental vacuity and complete incompetence of the deep stupor, just as slow movements in the partial stupors seem to represent a diluted inactivity reaction. This actual thinking disorder is not present in those forms of manic-depressive insanity which are characterized by elation, anxiety or depression but is seen only in stupors, occasionally in absorbed manic states (manic stupor) and sometimes in perplexity states. The psychological mechanisms of this last group are probably analogous to those of stupor, but this is not the place for a discussion of this topic.

Another associated symptom whose manifestations differ in depression and stupor is that of unreality. In the former there is frequently a feeling of unreality that is purely subjective, whereas the stupor case does not usually complain of this but does exhibit a difficulty in grasping the nature of his environment, which the typical depressive case never has.

[126]

The occurrence of other mood reactions than apathy in the same patient is also characteristic. Manic states (usually hypomanic) frequently occur during the phase of recovery from the stupor. This is an unusual, although not unknown, phenomenon in recovery from severe retarded depressions. The circular cases who swing from depression to elation usually show the milder types of depressive reaction which would never be confused with stupor. On the other hand, deep stupors very frequently are terminated by manic reactions, and if not by such means, recovery seems to occur merely in virtue of a gradual attenuation of the stupor symptoms. Rarely do we see a change to depression or anxiety heralding improvement. This tendency of the stupor reaction to remain pure or change to hypomania is a peculiarity which seems to put stupor in a class by itself among the manic-depressive reactions, as all the other mood reactions frequently change from one to the other.

Although apathy is the central pathognomonic symptom of stupor conditions, there are other mood anomalies to be noted. One of these is the tendency for inconsistency in, as well as reduction of, the expression of emotion. For instance, in the states where one would expect anxiety during the onset of stupor or in its interruptions, manifestation of this anxiety is often reduced to an expression of dazed bewilderment. In the anxiety states associated with stupor one does not meet with the restlessness and expressions of fear which would be ex [127] pected. Quite similarly, when a manic tendency is present, it occurs either in little bursts of isolated symptoms of elation (such as smiling or episodic pranks), or some of the evidences of elation which we would expect are missing. For instance, Johanna S. (Case 13) terminated her stupor with a hypomanic state which was natural except for her always wearing an expressionless face. Sometimes laughter occurs alone and gives the impression of a shallow affect, raising a suspicion of dementia præcox. In fact, such evidences of affect as do appear in the course of the stupor are apt to be isolated, queer and "dissociated." It does not seem as if the whole personality reacted in the emotion as it does in the other forms of manic-depressive insanity. For example, we may think of the resistiveness which is so frequently present when the patient seems in other respects to be psychically dead. One may recall the case of Meta S. (Case 15), who, otherwise inert, was occasionally seen with tears or smiles. Anna G. (Case 1), too, was often seen smiling or weeping. It was noted once of Charlotte W. (Case 12) that she ceased answering questions and remained immobile with fixed gaze, but when some mention was made of her going home she flushed and tears ran down her cheeks, although no change in the fixedness of her attitude or facial expression was seen.

When Johanna S. was visited by her daughter and was lying motionless in bed, she slowly extended her hands, apparently tried to speak, and then her eyes filled with tears. Two days [128] later, at the end of an interview when she had made a few replies, she settled down into her usual inactivity and, when further urged to answer, her eyes filled with tears. Similarly, too, in fairly deep stupor pin pricking may result in flushing, in tears or an increased pulse rate without the patient giving any other evidence of the stimulus being felt. These examples seem to show a larval effort at normal human response which, failing of complete expression, appeared as single isolated features of emotion suggesting true dissociation. We should also in this connection bear in mind the impulsive suicidal acts which occur either as unexpectedly as the impulsiveness in a true dementia præcox patient, or in a setting of coarse animal-like excitement that seems quite unrelated to the personality. One is reminded of the patient who made suicidal attempts during the period when she shouted like a huckster, giving no evidence whatever by her expression or the tone of her voice of feeling anxiety, sorrow or any other normal emotion.

All these queer and larval affective reactions remind one strongly of dementia præcox. The resemblance of the benign stupor to certain dementia præcox types is not merely a matter of identity with catatonic features (catalepsy, negativism). In these anomalous mood reactions it seems as if there were a definite dissociation of affect, and so there is. How then can we differentiate these emotional symptoms from the "dissociation of affect" which is regarded as a cardinal symptom of dementia præcox? [129] The answer is that this term is used too loosely as applied to the latter psychosis. It is a particular type of dissociation which is significant of the schizophrenic reaction, for in it there is an acceptance of what should be painful ideas evidenced either by incomplete manifestations of anxiety or depression or actually by smiling. We never see in dementia præcox the reverse—a painful interpretation of what would normally be pleasant. It is the pleasurable interpretation of what is really unpleasant that gives the impression of queerness in the mood of these deteriorating or chronic cases. In stupor, on the other hand, although this dissociation takes place, the mood is never inappropriate, merely incomplete in that all the components or the full expression of the normal reaction are not seen.

Our description of the mood reactions in stupor would be incomplete if we omitted to mention the occasional appearance of an emotional attitude not unlike that seen in many cases of involution melancholia, which reminds one in turn of the reactions of a spoiled child. The commonest of these manifestations is resistiveness that may occur when an examination is attempted, feeding is suggested, or a sanitary routine insisted upon. One also meets with resentfulness. One patient, who frequently showed this reaction, explained it retrospectively by saying that she wanted to be left alone. Quite analogous to this is sulkiness that occasionally appears. Then we have, particularly as recovery begins, other childish tricks, such as flippancy in answering ques [130] tions or the playing of pranks. Such tendencies naturally lead over to frank hypomanic behavior.

Finally, a peculiar characteristic of the stupor apathy must be mentioned. This is its tendency to interruptions, when the patient may return to life, as it were, for a few moments and then relapse. Such episodes occur mainly in milder cases or towards the end of long, deep stupors. It is interesting that the occasion for such reappearance of affect is frequently obvious. We usually observe them in response to some special stimulus, particularly something that seems to revive a normal interest. Visits of relatives are particularly common as such stimuli, in fact recovery can often be traced to the appearance of a husband, mother or daughter. It is also important to recognize that with this revived interest, other clinical changes may be manifest, that the thinking disorder may, for instance, be temporarily lifted. Helen M., for example, when visited by her mother was so far awakened as to take note of her environment, and remembered these visits after recovery like oases in the blank emptiness of her stupor. She further remembered that definite ideas were at such a time in her mind that ordinarily was vacant. She then had delusions of being electrocuted.

In summary, then, we may say that the *sine qua non* of the stupor reaction is apathy in all gradations, and that this apathy is as distinct a mood change as is elation, sorrow or anxiety. Incidental to this loss of affect there is a dissociation of emo [131] tional response whereby isolated expressions of mood appear without the harmonious coöperation of the whole personality which seems to be dead. Thirdly, there tends to be associated with the stupor reaction a tendency to childish behavior. Finally, the apathy and accompanying stupor symptoms may be suddenly and momentarily interrupted. An explanation of these apparently anomalous phenomena will be attempted in the chapter on Psychology of the Stupor Reaction.

[132]

CHAPTER VII
INACTIVITY, NEGATIVISM AND CATALEPSY

1. Inactivity. We must now turn our attention to the other cardinal symptoms of the stupor reaction, and quite the most important one of these is the inactivity. It is convenient to include under this heading both the reduction of bodily movement and the diminution or absence of speech. This inactivity is, of course, related to the apathy which we have just been discussing, in fact it is one of the evidences of the loss of emotion. We presume that a patient is apathetic when there is no expression in the face and when he does not respond to external stimuli, whether these be physical or verbal, by movement or by word.

Bodily inactivity is present in all degrees, and in some forty consecutive cases was recognizable in every one. In its most extreme form there is complete flaccidity of all the voluntary muscles, and relaxation of some sphincters. As a result of the latter we see wetting, soiling and drooling. Even those reflexes which are only partially under voluntary control, like those of blinking and swallowing, may be in abeyance; for instance, saliva may collect in the mouth because it is not swallowed, and [133] tube-feeding is frequently necessary on account of the failure of the patient to swallow anything that is put into his mouth. The eyes may remain open for such long periods of time that the conjunctiva and sclera may become quite dry and ulcerate. In these extreme cases there is, of course, no response to verbal commands. What is more striking, no reaction appears to pin pricks, so that it seems as if consciousness of pain were lost.

This deep torpor does not usually persist indefinitely. The commonest evidence of some form of consciousness persisting is probably to be seen in blinking when the eye is threatened or the sclera or cornea actually touched. A very large number of patients, when otherwise quite inactive, showed considerable response in their muscular resistiveness, the phenomena of which will be discussed shortly. The relaxation of the sphincters is apt to persist even after control of the rest of the body is exercised to the point of permitting the patient to stand or walk about.

The first phase of obvious conscious control is seen in those patients who will retain a sitting posture in bed or in a chair. The next stage is reached where the stuporous case can be stood upon his feet but cannot be induced to walk. The next degree is that of walking only when pushed or commanded. Finally spontaneous movement is observed in which the inactivity is evidenced merely by a great slowness.

No correlation can be established between restric [134] tions of speech and motion other than that present in the extremes. With complete inactivity there is almost always consistent mutism, and perfect freedom of speech does not, as a rule, appear until the movements are free. In between these extremes all variations are possible, even the deepest stupors are occasionally interrupted by one or two words; for instance, a patient may remain comatose, as it were, and absolutely mute for six months, then to every one's surprise say one or two words and relapse into a year of silence. Again one sees cases where movements have become fairly free and yet the patient says nothing. This is another example of that inconsistency in reaction which we have already noted in connection with the mood or affect.

In so far as inactivity is merely an expression of apathy, its causation will be considered in connection with the psychology of the stupor reaction as a whole. In so far as there may be specific factors, however, it may be of interest to consider what information the patients themselves give us from time to time as to what determined their inactivity. It is really surprising how frequently something can be gained either from careful notes taken during the stupor or from the retrospective accounts of the psychotic experiences. Of course when one considers the degree of amnesia which is usually present and the extent of the intellectual defect in general, it becomes obvious that one cannot think of getting anything like a complete explanation of the behavior of any given case. Nevertheless this material is [135] quite suggestive in the mass; it gives one some idea of the mental state as a whole.

Among 40 cases, 27 offered some explanation either during or following the psychosis. Of these, 20 spoke of feeling dead, numb or drugged, or feeling as if paralyzed or having lockjaw. This group, just half of all the cases, apparently ascribed their disability to something which seemed physical. One might call them somatopsychic cases. The other 7 gave more allopsychic explanations: 3 attributed their inactivity to outside influence; 3 more said they were afraid (one of these because she imagined herself to be in prison), which is analogous to the outside influence; the 7th case thought she would injure people if she moved.

The following are some examples of the statements of the somatopsychic group: Laura A.: "I can't move," and retrospectively, "My arms were stiff." Bridget B. claimed retrospectively that she felt dead or drugged, that her limbs were lifeless, she felt as if she had lockjaw. Johanna B. remembered being pricked with a pin on several occasions but claimed that she did not feel the pain at any time. This suggests a definitely hysterical mechanism. Anna L. (Case 16) said retrospectively that she felt as if she were dead, although walking around, and also that she thought she was a ghost and not supposed to speak. Anna M. said she had tried to speak but everything stuck in her throat. Alice R. said that she had no energy, did not want to talk. Meta S. (Case 15) claimed that while stupor [136] ous her tongue would not move. Isabella M. in intervals claimed that during the stuporous periods she felt as if dead and said retrospectively when the whole psychosis was over that it was "an effort to speak." Johanna S. (Case 13), while stuporous when pressed with questions would say: "I can't think," "I don't know," "I am twisted." When food was offered her she protested, "I am dead." Charlotte W. (Case 12), in reviewing her case, said: "I was mesmerized," "I thought I was dead." Anna G. (Case 1), in retrospect said: "I don't think I could speak," again "I made no effort," or "I did not care to speak." Henrietta H. (Case 8) said, "I lost speech." She claimed that she did not move because she was tired and had a numb feeling. Mary C. (Case 7) said that her tongue had been thick and that she felt dull. Rose Sch. (Case 6) said during the psychosis that her head was upside down and retrospectively that she had been mixed up, could not remember well, did not feel like talking. Mary D. (Case 4) said that she had been dazed, that she had not felt like talking, and that her limbs "were stiff like." We should probably also include here as a delusion of death the statement of Annie K. (Case 5) who wanted to die and thought she would do so if she kept still enough.

It is rather striking that among all the forty cases only one spoke of being sick—"I am so sick." Only one evaded questions with "that was my illness." One would expect a priori that these patients would offer some vague explanations or make complaints [137] of weakness. If these stupors were purely physical in origin, one would expect such explanations as weakness or illness to be offered in accounting for the inactivity. That there is a rather definite type of explanation offered is, we think, distinctly suggestive. If one tries to correlate and group the death ideas, one sees that they are all delusions of death or of loss of energy or complaints of hysterical symptoms that look like sham death. If the lack of energy complained of be looked upon as lifelessness, one can conceive of these explanations being variations of one theme, namely, that of death. In the last chapter it has been shown that a delusion of dying, being dead, or having been dead is extremely frequent in the stupor group. It would seem only natural then to regard the inactivity, in so far as it may be specifically determined, as an expression of some such delusion.

Psychiatrists are more or less aware of there being typical ideational contents in the different manic-depressive psychoses. For instance, every one is familiar with ideas of wickedness and inadequacy in depression, ideas of violence in anxiety, or expansive and erotic fancies in manic states. Quite similarly we have seen that death is a dominant topic in a stupor. Now in addition to these typical ideas we often hear expressed what we might term non-specific delusions, ideas that seem to have nothing to do with a peculiar type of reaction which the patient presents. It is therefore not surprising to [138] find that inactivity is not consistently ascribed to death or a related delusion.

For instance, Henrietta B. had much talk of higher powers that were controlling her, also said that it was fear which kept her quiet. Josephine G. said retrospectively that she had thought she would injure people if she moved and that if she opened her eyes she would murder the people around her. Johanna B. was afraid to talk because she fancied she was in prison. Laura A.: During her stupor was more vague, saying, "I can't move, they won't let me be," without betraying any suggestion of whom "they" might be. Finally Mary C. (Case 7) was still more indefinite, ascribing her immobility merely to fear. When one considers, however, that these five were the only ones who gave any atypical explanation of their inactivity among the thirty-seven cases, the preponderance of the death idea becomes striking.

2. Negativism. The next of the cardinal symptoms to be considered is negativism. This term, which is often loosely used, we would define as perversity of behavior which seems to express antagonism to the environment or to the wishes of those about the patient. Naturally it is only in the minor stupors that we see it in well-developed form as active opposition and cantankerousness. For example, Harriett C., who stood about until her feet became edematous, would spit out food when it was placed in her mouth but would eat if she were left alone with the food. Josephine G., in a milder state, [139] would turn her back on people. When more inactive once rolled out of bed and lay on the floor. At this time also she tried to keep people out of her room. Rarely, patients may have angry outbursts, as did Annie K. (Case 5) who would strike at the nurses.

Very often the failure to swallow and anomalous habits of excretion seem to be negativistic in their nature. One thinks at once of the necessity for tube-feeding, which is so common even when patients seem otherwise fairly active. Naturally this form of treatment is necessary only when the patient refuses to swallow. Quite frequently a refusal to urinate is met with so that catheterization is necessary, or a patient may never use the toilet when led to it, but will defecate or urinate so soon as he leaves it. These latter, like some other perversities, suggest reactions of a petulant, spoiled child.

By far the commonest manifestation is muscular resistiveness, often spoken of as "resistiveness." It was present in thirty-two out of thirty-seven of our cases. Usually it takes the form of a contraction of the whole system of voluntary muscles when the patient is touched or the bed approached. Often it appears only when any passive movement of the limb is attempted. All muscles of the limb then stiffen, making the member rigid. Sometimes the negativism is expressed by quite isolated symptoms, such as stiffness in the jaw muscles alone. One patient showed no opposition except by holding her urine for two days. Another kept her eyes constantly directed to the floor. The reaction of an [140] other showed no irregularity except for stiffness in the neck and arms and wetting herself once after she had been taken to the toilet. One displayed merely a slight stiffness in her arms. An interesting case was that of Annie G. (Case 1) who kept one leg sticking out of bed. If this were pushed in, she would protrude the other. Mary F. (Case 3) sometimes expressed her antagonism to the environment by slapping other patients. She spoke only twice in a year and a half, and each time it was when interfered with. By far the commonest cause of muscular movement in these inactive cases is resistiveness, and as a rule the inactivity is interrupted only by negativistic symptoms.

If we look for some explanation or correlation of these symptoms, we find that chance references to conduct seem to point in the same direction, namely, to the desire to be left alone. This resentment against interference again reminds us of the reactions of a spoiled child. For instance, Laura A., in manic spells during which she was still constrained and drooled, said, "I don't want to have my face washed." In the intervals she showed an intense muscular resistiveness. Mary G. used to say, "Leave me alone," and covered her head or buried it in the pillows. Maggie H. (Case 14) said in retrospect that she had wanted to be left alone. Similarly Alice R. thought she did not want to talk. Emma K. thought that she was in prison and apparently resented this. Henrietta B. combined in her behavior tendencies both to compliance and opposition. [141] When her arms were raised they retained the new position for a minute. Then she dropped them and said, "Stop mesmerizing me." But then she put them up again of her own accord, and when she had done this presented intense resistiveness to any movement. Later she extended her arms in front of her and said, "I am all right," in a theatrical manner, and then added, "Why don't you go away?"

There seems to be some correlation between inaccessibility and muscular resistiveness. For example, Charlotte W. (Case 12), whose condition varied a great deal, always lost the resistiveness when she became accessible, during which periods she also showed some facial expression. The resistiveness would invariably return when the inaccessibility reappeared. Caroline DeS. (Case 2) lost her resistiveness as she became more accessible, although the inactivity and apathy persisted. This tendency, which is quite common, suggests that muscular resistiveness represents a lower level of expression of opposition which patients put into words or purposeful actions when there is other evidence of some contact with the environment. Sometimes one observes both general resistiveness and specific acts. For instance, Mary G., who said, "Leave me alone," and covered her head or buried it in the pillows, accompanied her muscular resistiveness with laughter. This shows the affective nature of the apparently purposeless muscular tension. The case of Annie K. (Case 5) is more instructive. In the stage [142] of deeper stupor she had the automatic type of resistiveness but also outbursts of anger, particularly toward the nurses, striking one of them she said, "You are the cause of it all." When food was offered her, she said, "I wonder people would not leave me alone sometimes." Again, when her bed was approached, she would clutch and hold the bed clothes in an apparently aimless way as if the impulse to resist never reached its goal. Retrospectively she could not account for her muscular rigidity on the basis of definite ideas, and could recall only that she felt stubborn. In a later period when more accessible, she felt cross and did not want to be bothered. This emotional attitude was quite conscious with her, whereas the acts and speech of the earlier period, when her stupor was more profound, seemed more automatic and impulsive. In other words, the resistiveness looks like a larval attempt to express an idea which is probably not fully conscious and therefore gives the appearance of being aimless. As another example of this we may cite the case of Pearl F. (Case 9), who said when she recovered, "I was stubborn." In addition to the muscular resistiveness she had shown, she would often bite the bed clothes or scratch herself when she was approached. Mary F. (Case 3), while in a stupor, slapped at nearby patients quite aimlessly. When somewhat better, this conduct appeared in a more conscious form, as sullenness, indifference and smearing of feces (again the behavior of a naughty child). Here one might quote Laura A. once more, whose resis [143] tiveness when stuporous was intense but who in her manic spells expressed her negativism in a definite idea, "I don't want my face washed."

To summarize, then, we may say that negativism is apparently the result of a desire to be left alone, and that muscular resistiveness is a larval exhibition of the same tendency. But the appearance of this attitude in such aimless, impulsive acts or habits reminds us strongly of the dissociation of affect, which was commented on in the previous chapter. It would seem to be another example of this rather fundamental tendency of the stupor reaction, not merely to diminish conative reactions in general, but to reduce their appearance to that of isolated, partial and therefore rather meaningless expression.

3. Catalepsy. The last of the cardinal symptoms to be considered is catalepsy. It occurred in thirteen of thirty-seven cases, although it was present only as a tendency in three of these. If we define it as the maintenance of position in which a part of the body is placed regardless of comfort, we can see that sometimes it is difficult to differentiate from the phenomenon of resistiveness with its rigidity. It is most frequently observed in the hands and arms, perhaps because it is, as a rule, most convenient to demonstrate the retention of awkward positions in the upward extremities. But any part or even the whole body may be involved; for example, Charles O. retained standing positions even where balance was difficult. This phenomenon is often [144] accompanied by "waxy flexibility," where the joints move stiffly but retain whatever bend is given them, like a doll with stiff joints.

The significance of catalepsy is best studied by considering its relationship to other symptoms and by noting remarks made by the patients in reference to it. The most important observations which we have made seem to indicate that it never occurs with that degree of deep inactivity which suggests a complete lack of mentation on the part of the patient. One is therefore forced to conclude that back of this phenomenon there must be some purpose, some kind of an ideational content, although this may be of a primitive order. This is demonstrably true in some cases, at least such as that of Isabella M., who left her arm sticking up in the air but took it down to scratch herself and then put it back. Somewhat similarly, Charlotte W. (Case 12), when she was shown during convalescence a photograph of herself in a cataleptic state, said that that was when she was waiting to go to Heaven and was afraid to move. Again she remarked, "I was mesmerized." Josephine G., who showed only a tendency to catalepsy, said that she feared the devil would get control of those about her if she moved. Sometimes there is a development of this symptom from others which seem to be ideational in their origin. For instance, Charles O. began making flail-like movements. These passed over into slow circular motions which finally subsided into the maintenance of fixed position.

[145]

References to hypnotism are not infrequent, and in many cases there is evidence of a delusion that the posture is desired by those in charge of the patient. Annie G. (Case 1) said so directly. In retrospect she explained the holding of her arms in the air by saying, "I thought you wanted me to have them up." Henrietta B. at one examination kept her arms raised in the position in which they had been put for a minute and then dropped them, saying, "Stop mesmerizing me." But she then put them up again of her own accord and now presented intense resistance to any motion. Later she extended her arms in front of her and said, "I am all right," in a theatrical manner. Some patients give evidence in other symptoms of larval efforts at coöperation with the actual or supposed wishes of the physician and in such cases it is not impossible that passive movements are interpreted as orders. One must remember in this connection that the more primitive are the mental operations of any individual, the more important do signs, rather than speech, come to be a medium of communication with other people. As an example of this type we might mention Rose Sch. (Case 6), who flinched from pin pricks (showing that she felt them) but made no effort to get away. When somewhat clearer she said that she was "here to be cured." Similarly Mary D. (Case 4), who showed no catalepsy from ordinary tests, kept her head off the pillow for a long time after it was raised to have her hair dressed. She showed such perseveration in many constrained po [146] sitions. She too flinched from pin pricks but not only made no effort to prevent them but would even stick out her tongue to have a pin stuck in it.

The relationship of catalepsy to resistiveness is interesting but unfortunately complicated and unclear. In only one of our cases was catalepsy definitely present without resistiveness, and in one other a "tendency to catalepsy" was noted without muscular rigidity being observed. In this latter case, when the catalepsy became unquestionable, resistiveness also appeared. It is one thing to note this coexistence and another to explain it adequately. All that we can offer are mere speculations as to the real meaning of the association of these phenomena. It may be that the tension of muscles that occurs when resistiveness is present gives the idea to the patient of holding the position. There would be two possible explanations for this. We might think there is a dissociation of consciousness, like that of hysteria, where the feeling of tenseness in the muscles that comes from the resistance to gravity is not discriminated from the resistance to the movements made by the examiner. On the other hand, there might be a similar dissociation where the perception of contraction in the antagonistic muscles is interpreted as the action of the examiner in placing the limb in a given position. This latter view would seem, on the face of it, ridiculous, inasmuch as its presumes the existence of two directly opposed tendencies, namely, those of opposition to the will of the physician and compliance with it. But [147] ambivalent tendencies are frequently present in psychopathic states, and moreover we find occasionally some evidence in the behavior of the patient to substantiate this view. For example, at one stage of the stupor of Annie G. (Case 1), her arm could be moved without resistance. Then the elbow would catch and at this moment the position would be maintained. Such observation is highly suggestive of the resistance being signal for the catalepsy. In Isabella M. the catalepsy appeared when resistance to passive movements also developed. On the other hand, when the resistance became extreme, the catalepsy was reduced, and vice versa. This makes one think of two tendencies: suggestibility on the one hand, and opposition on the other. We might presume that when both are present and equally strong, stiffness with passive movements results as a kind of compromise, but when there is a greater development of one, the other is inhibited.

Such speculations remind one strongly of the psychology of conversion hysteria and of hypnotism. In some cases of stupor hysterical symptoms are quite definitely present. For instance, Celia G. began her psychosis with hysterical convulsions which would terminate with short periods of stupor. Later the stupor became persistent and during this stage she had catalepsy (and restiveness as well) in her left arm only. On recovery from her stupor she complained of stiffness in her hands, which examination proved to be a purely hysterical difficulty.

[148]

This whole subject is without question obscure and many more and very careful observations are needed before really satisfactory explanations can be given for these phenomena. That it is a reaction which is related to the primitiveness of the mental content and the intellectual deficit in stupor would seem to be a reasonable view, inasmuch as quite similar phenomena have been observed in a large number of animals, even among crustaceans. As a result of our own observations the only thing we feel at liberty to state with real confidence is that catalepsy is presumably a phenomenon mental in origin rather than somatic, because it always occurs in conditions which show other evidence of mentation.

Whatever may be the origin of the idea of the posture assumed, there can be little doubt that its indefinite maintenance is a phenomenon of perseveration. The conception of the position being in the patient's mind, it is easier to hold it than elaborate another idea. This, of course, is part of the intellectual disorder in stupor. In fact, it is difficult to imagine any one whose critical faculty was functioning coöperating in a test for catalepsy.

[149]

CHAPTER VIII
SPECIAL CASES: RELATIONSHIP OF STUPOR TO OTHER REACTIONS

We have described typical cases of benign stupor and isolated certain interrelated symptoms which, when they dominate the clinical picture, we believe establish the diagnosis of stupor, regardless of the severity of the reaction. These symptoms are apathy, inactivity, a thinking disorder and, quite as important as these, an absorbing interest in death. It is typical that the patient contemplates his dissolution with indifference or, at most, with mild or sporadic anxiety. There seems little reason to doubt that when these four symptoms occur alone, we are justified in making a diagnosis of stupor. The next problem is to consider the meaning and classification of cases where these symptoms occur in conjunction with others. This naturally introduces the subject of relationship of stupor to other manic-depressive reactions.

It is probably best to begin with presentation of three such cases.

Case 16.—*Anna L.* Age: 24. Admitted to the Psychiatric Institute August 21, 1916.

F. H. Maternal grandmother temporarily insane during illegitimate pregnancy, thereafter a little odd. Mother high strung [150] and emotional. Father high strung, impulsive and irritable.

P. H. As a child she was quick tempered, quite a spitfire and given to tantrums. At the age of 14 she became a vaudeville actress in Cleveland, which was the home of her childhood. When 17 she married a Jew, although she was herself a Catholic. Her husband noted that she was fretful, sensitive, resentful and quick tempered, although apt to recover quickly from her rages. Previously healthy, neurotic symptoms began with marriage, taking the form of stomach trouble and a tendency to fatigue. Shortly after marriage an abortion was induced. After being married for two years she had a quarrel and separated from her husband. They were reconciled later, but in the meantime she had been having relations with another man. When 20 an abdominal operation was performed in the hope of relieving her gastric symptoms, but no improvement occurred. The patient after recovery stated that she continued to be nervous, shaky and dizzy, at times trembling when going to bed at night. Two years later, however, she took up Christian Science and showed objectively some improvement in her health, although according to her later accounts she continued to feel somewhat nervous and fatigable. Her husband stated that at this time she also began to ponder much about such questions as the difference between life and death, what "matter" was, and also studied "grammar" and "etiquette." According to the patient some five or six months before admission she began to have peculiar sensations following intercourse — a feeling of bulging in the arms, legs and back of the neck. One evening after an automobile ride there were peculiar sensations on her right side like "electricity" or as if she were inhaling an anesthetic. She gasped and thought she was dying. Two months before her admission she went with her husband and his family to a summer resort where she felt increasingly what had always been a trouble to her, namely, the nagging of this family.

Just before her breakdown, because she went daily to the Christian Science rooms in order to avoid the family, they suspected her of immorality and accused her of going to meet other men. Even her husband began to question her motive. Retrospectively the patient herself said that she now felt she was losing her mind and did not wish to talk to any one. At the time she [151] told her husband that she felt confused and as if she were guilty of something and being condemned. Repeatedly she said she knew she was going to get the family into a lot of trouble. Once she spoke of suicide, and for a while felt as if she were dying. Finally she became excited and shouted so much that she was taken to the *Observation Pavilion*, where she was described as being restless and noisy, thinking that she was to be burned up and that she had been in a fire and was afraid to go back.

On admission she looked weary and seemed drowsy. Questions had to be repeated impressively before replies could be obtained, when she would rouse herself out of this drowsy state. She seemed placid and apathetic. She said that nothing was the matter, but soon admitted that she had not been well, first saying that her trouble was physical and then agreeing that it had been mental. When asked whether she was happy or sad, she said "happy," but gave objectively no evidence of elation. Her orientation was defective. She spoke of being in New York and on Blackwell's Island, but could not describe what sort of place she was in, saying merely that it was "a good place," or "a nice country place," again "a good city." Once when immediately after her name L. had been spoken and she was asked what the place was, she said "The L." She knew that she had arrived in the hospital that day but said that she had come from Cleveland, and to further questions, that she had come by train, but she could not tell how she reached the Island. She claimed not to know what the month was and guessed that the season was either spring or autumn (August). She gave the year as 1917, called the doctor "a mentalist," and the stenographer "a tapper," or "a mental tapper." She twice said she was single. When asked directly who took care of her, said "Mr. Marconi," who she claimed at another time had brought her to the hospital. To the question, who is he? she replied, "Wireless," and could not be made to explain further. That night she urinated in her bed, and later lay quite limp, again held her legs very tense.

For five days she remained lying quietly in bed for the most part, although once she called out "Come in, I am here," "Jimmie, Jimmie" (husband's name). Several times she threw her bed clothes off. Otherwise she made no attempt to speak and took insufficient food unless spoon-fed. At one examination she looked up rather dreamily but did not answer. When shaken she [152] breathed more quickly and seemed about to cry but made no effort to speak. When left to herself she closed her eyes and did not stir when told she could go back to the ward. She was then lifted out of her chair and took a step or two and stopped. Such urging had to be repeated, as she would continue to remain standing, looking about dreamily, although finally when taken hold of she whimpered. When she got to the dining-table she put her hand in the soup and then looked at it. So far there is nothing in this case atypical of what we would call a partial stupor. The cardinal symptoms of apathy, inactivity, with a thinking disorder, are all present and dominate the clinical picture. There is, further, the history of a delusion of death during the onset of the psychosis. Had her condition remained like this, there would be no difficulty in classifying the case, but other symptoms appeared.

Five days after admission she was restless, somewhat distressed, and announced that she wanted to talk to the physician. When examined, the distress, with some whimpering, continued. She asked the doctor not to be harsh to her, frequently said there was something wrong and began to cry. A normal interest appeared only once, when she spontaneously said she wanted to see her relatives. A most interesting feature, however, was a certain perplexity that now appeared. She spoke of this directly: "I do not know what it is all about. I know you are a doctor, that is all. I don't know whether I passed out and came back again or what—I don't know what to make of it." She also felt confused about her marriage—"There is where all the mixup is. I was married when I was 16." She was reminded that she had said she was single, and replied "I am single." Then where is your husband? she was asked. "He must be dead." She recalled the examination on admission and remembered some of the questions that she was asked then, also knew that she had been at the Observation Pavilion and that she had reached this hospital by boat. On the other hand she still claimed that the year was 1917, and in connection with the delusion of having died was quite unclear as to the time. She said that it seemed as if she had died many years ago and that she had come to the hospital years ago. She also spoke of having died at a summer resort the year before. When asked for her age, she said that she must be very [153] old, but on the other hand claimed that she was supposed to die and to come to the hospital when she was 26 (two years more than her actual age).

Her psychosis continued from then on for about ten weeks. She soon began to feed herself, but otherwise for most of this period remained quietly in bed, looking about a good deal, although showing no particular mood reaction until questioned, when she was apt to make repeated statements about her perplexity—that she did not know what it was all about, every one had mixed her up, everything was so strange, "my head is mixed up, I am trying to straighten things up." She frequently when interviewed became lachrymose and often with her subjective confusion there was considerable anxiety. Another unusual phenomenon for a stupor patient was that she was frightened at a thunder storm. On the whole, however, her apathy and indifference were quite marked. For instance, during the latest phase of her psychosis, when the nurses would sometimes make her dance with them, she did so but without showing any interest and not until immediately before her recovery did she begin to speak spontaneously to any extent whatever. A marked difference from the ordinary stupor was that this apathy was invariably broken into when she was questioned and ideas came to her mind, the nature of which seemed to be essentially connected with her perplexity.

Not only did ideas appear more frequently than one meets them in stupor cases, but they were present in greater variety. The dominant stupor death idea was, it is true, almost constantly present, but it did not come to the direct and unequivocal expression which we are accustomed to see in typical stupor. She did not say "I am dead," or "I was dead," but it was always "It seems as if I were dead," or "I think I must have died," or some such dubious statement. Other ideas were that her mother was dead and had been put into a box. She frequently gave her maiden name and said that she lived in Cleveland with her mother and that this was Cleveland. At times she thought she was engaged and was going to be married to her husband shortly. Again there were notions that her husband had married somebody else or that some harm was going to come to him. Sometimes [154] she thought that her mother's name was her own, that is, Mrs. L. The hospital once seemed like a convent to her.

Her subjective and objective confusion seemed quite definitely to be connected with the insecurity and changeability of these ideas. It appeared as if insight and delusion were struggling for mastery in her mind, so that reality and fancy were alternately, even simultaneously, possessing her, and that this gave her the feeling of perplexity from which she suffered. Once when she remarked "It seems as if I had been dead all the time," she was questioned more about this and replied, "Well, sometimes I thought I was dead, at other times it seemed as if I wasn't." In answer to a direct question about her feeling of confusion she said "I don't know. I know I have lots of good friends, they all want to help me and it seems as if everything got mixed up between the L.'s (her married name) and the G.'s (her maiden name)." This was apparently an elaboration of the wavering ideas she had about her singleness or her married state. Once after referring to her husband as her sweetheart whom she was to marry, and immediately thinking that perhaps he had married somebody else, she added, with a sigh, "The more this goes on, the more mixup." In short, any question, even on some apparently neutral topic, seemed to start up conflicting ideas in her mind, the inconsistency of which she recognized without being able to control their appearance. Hence, whenever she was spoken to, she became perplexed and distressed.

Her orientation gradually improved so that, although it remained vague, it was no longer glaringly inaccurate. Then quite suddenly she one day came to a nurse and asked how long she had been in the hospital. When told, she remarked that it seemed as if she had spent the whole winter there. She was examined at once and found to be quite clear and at first in good control of her faculties. She remembered a good many of her ideas, in fact was able to elaborate a little from memory on what had already been reported from her utterances during the psychosis. The recovery was not immediately complete, however, for at this examination, when told that she had constantly given her maiden name, she became distressed and said the physician was trying to mix her up and was reluctant for this reason to discuss her ideas. This soon passed, however, and within a few days she [155] was quite normal and had remained so for some months after her discharge from the hospital, when last seen. In fact, according to the husband, she was in better mental and physical health following the psychosis than she had been for years.

Essentially, then, this case shows what was at first a typical partial stupor, but soon became complicated by a tendency for questioning to provoke rather a free flow of ideas and a distressed perplexity. This symptom of perplexity soon grew to dominate the clinical picture, so that the psychosis was really a perplexity ushered in by a brief stupor reaction with a background of stupor symptoms running through it. The second case shows similar tendencies but different from the one whose history has just been cited in that the perplexity was never complained of by the patient herself and that her emotional reactions were more marked and varied.

Case 17.—*Celia C.* Age: 18. Admitted to the Psychiatric Institute May 2, 1914.

F. H. Four years after this attack her mother was a patient in the hospital with an atypical manic-depressive psychosis from which she apparently recovered.

P. H. The patient herself was described by superficial observers as being bright, sociable, well-informed and very ambitious.

When 18 years of age she was working very hard preparing for some examinations, and worried lest she should fail in them. Some years later the patient accounted for her psychosis by saying she had a quarrel with her sister, immediately after which she began to feel depressed. The anamnesis states that she was slow, complained of not being able to think and feeling as if she had no brain. She was sent to a general hospital, where she was apprehensive, wanted her mother to stay with her and one night called out "Mother."

[156] The case being recognized after a few days as a psychosis, she was sent to the *Observation Pavilion*, where she was described as jumping about in bed in a jerky, purposeless manner, resistive when anything was done for her, and mute. Her sister reported that when she visited her the patient said "Go away, I am dead."

On admission she looked dazed, stared vacantly and had a tendency to draw the sheet over her. When put on her feet she let herself fall limply. At times she became agitated, sobbed and cried loudly, especially when attempts were made to examine her physically, or, when she was asked questions, she scarcely spoke.

Her psychosis lasted but a little more than three months under observation and was characterized by the following symptoms: She was usually in bed, staring blankly or appearing otherwise quite indifferent and apathetic, but not infrequently, especially during the first few weeks, she was quite restless, resistive, whined and suddenly appeared startled or distressed with no occasion for this reaction in the environment. Rarely she was suddenly assaultive. When attempts were made to examine her, she was frequently mute or would repeat the question with a rising inflection, not getting anywhere, or would say, "What shall I say," or "I, I — —" never finishing her sentence. After orientation questions she might say "This is — this is — this is — —" all this, together with a rather perplexed appearance, gave the impression of considerable bewilderment, but at no time did she complain of autopsychic perplexity. It was difficult to judge of her orientation on account of her failure to answer questions, but it soon appeared that she knew the names of the nurses, for she sometimes called them spontaneously by name. She always ate reluctantly.

During these examinations, however, other symptoms often appeared. When she was talked to, she was apt to indulge in depressive statements and show considerable distress. Such remarks were: "I must confess my guilt," "I am a bad girl and I have to face my guilt," or "I have sinned," or, standing up with a dramatic air, "I must stand up and tell the truth." Once she said, "It is too late to live now." She spoke of having lied and usually would not say what about, but once on questioning replied "I said I would not tell what happened here." She was asked, [157] What do you mean? and answered "I took my oath not to tell anything." Pressed further she said that the nurses poisoned her. Another time she said she was in prison. To her aunt who visited her she said, "I am a prostitute," and once she remarked to the doctor, "I have killed my honor," and on another occasion in the middle of the night she called out, "Chinatown Charlie, come here." She thought the doctor was her brother.

Most of these statements were associated with painful emotion, but there were a few occasions when an element of elation cropped out. Thus on one occasion she laughed, another time gripped the doctor's pad and tried to read it. When the nurse laughed, she made a funny grimace at her and said "Why do you laugh?" Again she once sang two songs, but after the first verse got stuck and kept repeating one word.

At the end of three months she improved rather rapidly and was in a condition for discharge as "recovered" a month later. Retrospectively she said that she recalled feeling guilty, thinking that her mother was dead, having been killed by the patient as a result of worrying over the latter's failure in her examinations and refusal to eat. She remembered, too, that at times she thought the building was burning. Some things like "Chinatown Charlie" she denied remembering, although she had a good recollection for the external facts throughout the psychosis. Her insight was superficially good, but she was reluctant to discuss her psychosis, in fact claimed that she had been made more of a lunatic by coming to the hospital than she was on admission.

Some five years later she had another somewhat similar attack, again following a quarrel, this time with a fellow employee. In this second psychosis, however, manic elements were much more prominent.

Here again, then, we have the symptoms of apparent apathy, inactivity, and similar ideas of death, but the thinking disorder was possibly not very profound, inasmuch as she had a good memory for external events. Her ideas, too, are much more florid than those which we customarily meet with in stupor cases, but the most marked peculiarity was [158] that this "stupor" was liable to constant interruption, either spontaneously or as a result of questioning, which always produced a mood reaction. She was apathetic only so long as she was left alone. In other words, whenever an effort was made to test what seemed to be apathy, the evidences of it disappeared.

The third case to be considered is somewhat like that of the first, Anna L. (Case 16), in that with the inactivity and apathy there was a coincident subjective perplexity. The apathy, however, was less marked than in the case of Annie L.

Case 18. — *Catherine M.* Age: 24. Admitted to the Psychiatric Institute November 10, 1913.

F. H. Information as to the family is confined to the two parents. The mother, who was frequently seen, seemed to be a natural, sensible woman. The father, on the other hand, had been alcoholic all his life, had had two convulsions while drinking, and had little respect from any member of the family, including the patient.

P. H. The patient was said always to have been healthy, from a physical standpoint, although never robust. She got on well at school, and then worked first as a stock girl and later as clerk in a department store, where her work was efficient and she advanced steadily. As a child she played freely with other girls but little with boys. As she grew older she moved about socially a little more, made the acquaintance of men as well as of girls, but never cared much for the former and had no love affairs until she met her husband. She was never demonstrative but always rather quiet and modest. Occasionally she spoke of thinking that people talked about her, but the informant doubted if she brooded over this, because she was not of a worrying disposition. Considering the ideas which appeared in her psychosis, it is striking that in her normal life she was rather [159] antagonistic towards her father on account of his alcoholism and the crudity of his speech and manners.

When she met her husband she liked him from the first, although she at no time became really demonstrative. They were engaged for a year, during which time she agreed to a postponement of three months for the marriage, which was suggested by her mother. For some time before this event she was working harder than usual and seemed a bit worn out. She ceased working a month before marriage and improved physically, although she became rather nervous, that is, she was more easily startled, an accentuation of what had been a characteristic for some years. Her husband stated that at this time she became fearful of the approaching marriage relations and asked him to be kind to her in this respect. She was married a year before admission. For two and a half months she refused intercourse and visited her mother's home a great deal. She finally submitted. She was quite frigid but became pregnant at once. Her abnormality then became apparent. She kept the fact of her pregnancy to herself for several months and then when she told her mother wanted to have an abortion performed. Neurotic symptoms appeared. She became sensitive with her husband, correcting his grammar, and cried easily. She also began to be anxious about the approaching childbirth, and with this became more religious.

For the first few days after the delivery, she was fussy with the nurse so that two in succession had to be discharged. On the fifth day she woke up and seeing a nurse lying on the couch beside her bed thought the latter was colored. On the seventh day she had a dream in which she thought she "nearly died in childbirth." Then she began to talk of dying for her baby or of having two babies, of dying herself and rising again after Easter Sunday. She became antagonistic to her husband and with this excited and confused so that she was taken to the Observation Pavilion.

On *admission* she looked pale and exhausted, had a slight temporary fever and a coated tongue. Her orientation was usually vague but sometimes she gave fair answers. Her verbal productions were rather fragmentary and with the exception of some repetitions there did not seem to be any special topics which dominated her train of thought.

[160] For some days the great weakness and the slight fever continued, and then, as it gradually cleared up, there came a change in her mental condition that settled into the state which characterized the rest of her psychosis. She talked less and was often quite inactive, frequently lying with her eyes closed for long periods, or sat or stood about. Such movements as she made were slow and languid. Her expression was either blank, absorbed, or gave the appearance of peculiar appealing perplexity. This last was not infrequently associated with a rather sheepish smile. She was never resistive and always ate and slept well. With the exception of a few times she did not soil herself. The most interesting feature of her mood reaction was that in a general setting of a slight perplexity there appeared at times and evidently associated with definite ideas, changes in her emotional state. Sometimes this was a matter of distress or of mild ecstasy, sometimes she became markedly blocked. There was at no time any frank elation, but often an appropriate smile, that is, appropriate to the situation and to the thought to which she was giving expression at the time. Then, rarely, there were sudden bursts of peculiar conduct, such as throwing herself on the floor or running down the hall. When questioned as to her motive for these acts, she would flush, look perplexed and apparently be unable to explain them.

Her verbal productions dealt with a rather limited range of topics which can be briefly summarized. As in the other cases, the reader will notice that the bulk of these ideas are of a kind not usually prominent in the typical stupor cases. Many of her thoughts seemed centered around her husband. She always knew him when he visited her, but in her thoughts there was a constant change as to his personality. She persistently confused him with the physicians, with her father, and with God, and one remark is typical, "I thought he was God, priest, doctor, lawyer—well, I wanted to go to Heaven; I thought he would still be my husband; I always hoped that I would be home in Heaven." Not unnaturally with this confusion there were doubts about her marriage. People said her marriage was wrong and her husband bad. Frequently she thought he was dead, or voices informed her that she was not married to him, or that he was the devil in Hell. In this connection she also said that people called her a [161] whore, or it seemed as if she were accused of not being married.

As prominently as appeared the ideas of the invalidity or impossibility of her marriage, to the same extent did her father assume an important rôle for her. As a rule he appeared in religious guise as God, but often he was the doctor—"I knew my father at home and my father in Heaven; which God do you mean? did you say God or father?" At times she spoke of being in Heaven and that God seemed to be God, doctor or priest. In this connection there were ideas of being under the power of some one, God, devil or father.

As is usually the case where strong interest is expressed in the father, ideas of the mother being dead occurred, although in the frankest form she reported them as dreams; for instance, one night she woke up screaming, said that she had dreamed that her mother was dead and her sister dying. That, in the psychoanalytic sense, this represented a removal of a rival, making union with her father easy, appeared in the statement that her father was dead but that she had dreamed he had come to life again for some one else. When asked what she meant, the question had to be repeated several times, then she said "My mother died, my father and mother had a quarrel." There is more than a suggestion here of a difference in the significance of death, in so far as it concerned the two parents. The mother dies and remains dead, that is, she is gotten rid of. The father dies but takes on a spiritual existence and comes to life again, a frequent method in psychoses for legitimizing the idea of union with the parent by elimination of the grossly physical.

There were strikingly few allusions to the plainly sexual. She spoke of being married to the doctor, and even went so far as to say that they belonged together in bed. On another occasion she called him "darling." Once she reported that it was said that she was going to have babies and babies and babies. These references were, however, quite isolated, so that the erotic formed a very small part of her productions.

Delusions of death, we have seen, are the most constant content of true stupors. In this case they were present but distinctly in the background. She spoke quite frequently of being in Heaven. She also talked of being crucified. Once she said "I [162] died but I came back again." This last utterance was rather significant in that frankly accepted ideas of death were unusual; for instance, she would say sometimes, "I think I am in Heaven, again not. It confuses me, but I know I am in Heaven."

In general, then, her ideas were, on the whole, not at all typical of stupor but much more like those met with in other manic-depressive conditions. Correlated with this was an unusual mood picture. Quietness and apparent apathy of the patient were interrupted by little bursts of emotion, and throughout the psychosis there was a coloring of perplexity. Not only was this last objectively noticeable, but she spoke very frequently of it and always in connection with the inconsistency of the ideas in her mind which puzzled her. For instance, in speaking to the doctor she said "I think of you as Bill (her husband's name) sometimes—I get confused thinking of Bill as God, doctor, lawyer, priest." Again, referring to her husband, she made these curious statements: "They seemed to speak of him as being in the wrong—the right—it seems that the right devil is the wrong one for me—they say he is not the right one for me; they say he went wrong from the time we were married." Again, she said that she did not know who her father was, and went on: "It puzzles me, this father business, I knew my father at home and my father in Heaven." Again, "Which God do you mean? Did you say God or father?" A hint as to how this subjective confusion made the environment seem uncertain comes from the statement, "You looked like the devil and yet you were God."

Distress and anxiety appeared not infrequently and always appropriately. The distress was usually occasioned by an idea of injury to others, as when she cried over the fancied accusation of drowning her husband and mother; or in connection with accusations of herself, such as when she reported "They called me a whore." As has been stated, there was never any frank elation, but an element of pleasurable expansive emotion was frequently present in connection with her religious utterances. This came particularly when she spoke of union with her father as God. She seemed to swell with ecstatic emotion. It was especially well marked once when she threw herself on the floor and when asked what she was trying to do replied, "I want to do what God wants me to do, drop dead or anything at all." [163] Perhaps the most unusual affective reaction was a blocking which occurred when certain topics appeared. This is a phenomenon quite unusual for stupor, where speech seems to stimulate and arouse the patient as a rule. One got the impression that ideas tended to come into this patient's mind which were painful enough to disturb her capacity for connected thought. A good example of this reaction was when she was speaking of her father having died and coming to life again. On being asked what she meant, she became quite blocked and the question had to be repeated several times, when finally the apparently unrelated statements appeared: "I dreamed my mother died—they had a quarrel." Who had a quarrel? she was asked, and replied "My mother and father." Apparently her thinking about her father coming to life for some one not her mother stimulated deeply unconscious ideas concerning the separation of her mother and father, and her taking the mother's place, and these ideas were sufficiently revolutionary to upset her capacity of speech for the time being.

She recovered completely about six and a half months after her admission.

If we consider together the common features of these three cases, we see that they resemble stupors only in the presence of inactivity and apparent apathy. It is true that death appears in the ideational content but not with that prominence, bordering on exclusiveness, which characterizes such delusions in the true stupors. These three patients give one the impression of being absorbed in thoughts that have many variations. It seems as if they had difficulty in grasping the facts of the environment, while feeling at the same time the vividness of the changing internal thoughts, hence a confusion develops which is either subjective, objective, or both. [164] It is probably the introversion of attention which gives rise to the apparent apathy, because normal emotions emerge as part of our contact with reality around us. This lack of contact with the environment leads also to inactivity. If one's attention and interest is turned inwards, there can be no evidence of mental energy exhibited until the patient is roused to contact with the people or things about him. It is noteworthy that in these cases emotional expression emerged when the patients were stimulated to some productiveness in speech.

These conditions really constitute a different psychosis in the manic-depressive group, essentially they are perplexity states such as have recently been described by Hoch and Kirby. [7] Not infrequently we see exhibitions of this tendency in what are otherwise typical stupors. For example, Mary F. (Case 3) (the third case to be described in the first chapter), showed for a few days after admission a condition when she was essentially somewhat restless in a deliberate aimless way. At the same time she looked dazed or dreamy. With this restlessness she appeared at times "a little apprehensive." Although she spoke slowly, with initial difficulty she answered quite a number of questions. Her larval perplexity was evidenced by the doubt expressed in a good many of her utterances, such as, "Have I [165] done something?" "Do people want something?" "I have done damage to the city, didn't I?" When asked what she had done, she said, "I don't know." She asked the physician, "Are you my brother?" and when questioned for her orientation said, "Is not this a hospital?" The atmosphere of perplexity also colored the information which she did recall correctly; for instance, when asked her address, she said, "Didn't I live at — —?" then giving the address correctly.

As stated in Chapter V dealing with the ideational content of stupor, one has to look on the delusions of patients as symptoms subject to analysis and classification just as truly as the variations in mood or intellectual processes, in fact they should be subject to the same correlation as are the mental anomalies which are usually studied, particularly if we are to understand these psychoses as a whole. Let us, therefore, consider the death ideas in the three cases studied in this chapter. We find that, as in the ordinary stupors, there are delusions of death, also of mutual death (with the father), but there is a tendency to elaboration so that the death is only part of a larger Œdipus drama, the rest of which is usually lacking in stupors. Here it is present. So we have thoughts of the death of the mother or husband, another rival, considerable preoccupation with Heaven, and also erotic fancies.

We find in manic-depressive insanity a tendency for more or less specific ideational contents with dif [166] ferent types of the psychoses. [8] For example, there are religious and erotic fancies or ambitious schemes dominating the thoughts of manic patients, fears of aggression and injury met with in anxiety cases, and so on. In stupors, death seems to be a state of non-existence with other meanings lacking or only hinted at occasionally. When it tends to be elaborated, it leads over to formulations suggesting personal attachments and emotional outlet, and then we are apt to find interruptions of the pure stupor picture. For example, Charlotte W. (Case 12), whose case has been described, thought much about being in Heaven and ended with a hypomanic state. Atypical symptoms appear just as constantly in these cases, as do the atypical ideas. In other words, the thought content is definitely correlated with the clinical picture.

As the clinical pictures show the relationship of stupor to other psychoses, so there is also a correlation with varying formulations of the death fancy. We are now in a position to define more narrowly what death means in stupor. It is an accepted fact, a Nirvana state. When death means union with God or appears in other religious guise, manic symptoms tend to develop. When it is unwelcome and appears as "being killed," we find anxiety symptoms. A patient can conceive of death variously and have [167] various clinical pictures. A knowledge of the metamorphoses of ideas and their relationship to other symptoms enables us to understand such cases, that, without this key, seem confused and lawless jumbles of symptoms. Such theories tend to justify the view of essential unity of the manic-depressive group.

It would be instructive at this point to consider another case which illustrates beautifully how a stupor reaction may crystallize out of other manic-depressive states when attention has become focused on personal death. This patient went through four phases while under observation. First, while showing a perplexed expression but with fair orientation, she gave utterance to erotic and expansive fancies. She was restless, somewhat intractable and gave the impression of brooding over her imaginations rather than luxuriating in them. In other words, her condition seemed to be more that of absorbed than active mania. Second, these same ideas, somewhat reduced, continued in an apathetic state while impulsive symptoms developed: She began to shout like a huckster to be taken to Heaven and made numerous affectless, suicidal attempts. Third, came a true stupor and, fourth, a period of recovery when the stupor symptoms all disappeared but insight into the falsity of her ideas was lacking.

Case 19.—*Celia H.* Age: 19. Admitted to the Psychiatric Institute October 22, 1913.

F. H. The father was living; he always drank, and especially in later years contributed little to the support of the family. [168] The mother was living and said to be normal, while a brother was coincidentally insane, with a recoverable psychosis.

P. H. The mother stated that the patient was bright at school, enjoyed company and going out, had a droll wit, was not at all seclusive, no dreamer, helped to support the family and was efficient. She was very much attached to her brother and once said that if anything should ever happen to him she thought she would die. She also cared much for her older sister, with whom she worked, and for her mother.

Three months before the patient's admission her brother became depressed, mute, seemed worried, cried at times. He was sent to the country. Two months before admission, when the mother and the patient went to bring the brother to town, and while they were at the station, he suddenly tried to throw himself under a train but was restrained just in time. The patient appeared intensely frightened, but did not talk. In fact, she seemed somewhat bewildered and at once became dull. "Her movement and manner were much as at present."

When the patient was able later to give a retrospective account of the onset, she claimed that for some months before this incident she saw that her brother was losing his mind. She worried about this as well as about her work, and felt worn out. She said that when the brother tried to throw himself under the train she was terrified and could not speak or move, and that her mind got upset at once, "I lost my memory." The others forgot her and left her alone on the platform. Strangers put her on another train and she knew nothing until she arrived at home.

The mother added that at the time when the incident with the brother happened, the patient was menstruating and that this ceased at once.

At home she sat about inactive and did not seem even to worry. Whenever any one asked her about her brother she replied that he was dead. For two weeks before admission she said she was rich, that she owned all the property around. She also said she was married to Mattie S. In this connection the mother says that a foolish neighborwoman, the mother of Mattie S., told the patient since her sickness, by way of encouragement, that she should marry her son (the man mentioned). Finally, the patient [169] also expressed the idea that her mother was a stranger, that her real mother was dead.

At the *Observation Pavilion* she was described as wandering about in a perplexed manner, restless, resistive, answering few questions and in a low tone. She said things were "changed," also that she was married to S.

Under Observation: 1. For about ten days the patient's condition may be described as follows: The most striking feature was a certain restlessness with insistence on going out, with complaints that this and that had been done to her and with senseless struggling when interfered with. But all the motions were slow, the whole restlessness aimless and impulsive. Although the facial expression was somewhat perplexed, it changed remarkably little, and whenever asked whether she felt worried or anxious she denied it, and, indeed, there was only a suggestion of perplexity in her face.

The ideas which she expressed during this time referred to a few topics only, namely, marriage, wealth, and State prison. The remarkable fact was that all the ideas about marriage and wealth were spoken of, often immediately, again after some interval, now in the positive and again in the negative sense. Thus she said she was "Mrs. S.," again "You kept me from marrying Mattie S.," or "I am not supposed to be here—I am a married person," but also "You kept me from getting married." Or, "Take off that black dress, I am a bride," again "You have taken my bridal crown off my head," "The steamboats (seen from the window) are mine—I own the ships, the oceans, the land and everything," or again, she said she owned a kingdom, was Sh.'s wife, a wealthy woman, had millions. Sometimes she connected the millions with Sh. "Sh. has millions." On the other hand, she said: "I owned all this before I came. I have nothing now," or "You have taken the regal crown from me," "You have made a pauper of me," "They did it again, they took my millions away," or "Let me out, they are taking my millions."

Other ideas throughout this period were that this was a State prison, that "bums" were around. On one occasion she said "You can't put down all these things and make me out a lunatic." At another time she pulled a patient's hair and then said without fun: "I fixed the leading lady of the dump—she knows a lot, [170] but she does not know enough to keep her soup cool." When questioned about this woman (who at the time while cleaning had moved the furniture), she said: "I don't know where I am at."

The orientation during these days was not markedly disordered, when one got down to it. Although she spoke of State prison, it was always found she knew the name and the location of the hospital, the names of people around her, even the date approximately, though she was apt to say it was February 19, 1492, or October 19, 1492, or when the year was not given as 1492 she said it was "1900 or 1901, or 1911 or 1912." Frequently, however, it was hard to hold her attention.

Finally, it should be mentioned that she very often wet herself in bed or when standing, even when standing in the examining room.

2. The period following and lasting for two months may be given in the form of abstracts of each note.

November 7: Yesterday quiet, though struggling. Says without change of expression, "I saw four people killed—my mother, my brother, a priest, and my dear sister—we were all killed." Again, "I don't know where I am," "I am an orphan, my people died" (without affect).

November 20: More quiet recently, says little, but tries to get out when brought to the examining room, but when not prevented walks slowly about as before, says she wants to go home. Looks peculiarly blank.

November 23: Has remained quiet, says she is Dr. M.'s wife. But when told she is not married, she agrees. Her attitude towards the doctor is not changed, but when the nurses talk to him, she has tried to prevent it.

December 6: Has remained quietly in bed, gazing about. Slow in motion. She has spoken of being Dr. M.'s wife, again President Wilson's wife, again "Vincent (brother) is the ruler of the world."

At interview says little, seems abstracted, answers briefly in low tone. (Does anything bother you?) "No." (Are you natural?) "Yes." (Who are you?) "C. H." (correct). (You said you were the President's wife?) "No." (Are you married?) "No." (You talked about the kingdom?) "I own the kingdom" (affectlessly). (Where is Vincent?) "Here." (Have you heard [171] him?) "Yes." (What did he say?) "Nothing." (Is he all right?) "Yes." (Where is your mother?) "Home." (Why don't you go home?) "I can't." (Why not?) "I can't." (Why not?) "The family tree is broken, the Cardinal." (What about him?) "Nothing." (Retrospectively she said later she thought her brother was a cardinal.)

December 8: When her mother visited her she said "It is about time you come—I thought you were dead." Has walked down the hall "looking" for her dead cousin. When asked if she wanted to see her brother, said, "Ain't he dead?"

December 12: Cries out in an affectless tone like a huckster, "Father MacN., take me to Heaven," repeating this over and over.

December 15: Quiet as a rule, then for a time at the door, pulling at it and with whining voice but affectlessly saying "Give me the key— I want to go to the river—you can't keep me from Heaven—it is either Heaven or the river, give me the keys, give me the keys, open the door," "The niggers are taking possession." To the physician to whom she had claimed to be married, often repeats "You don't belong to me, I don't belong to you." (What about the niggers?) "A band of niggers, that is all they are." (Are the nurses niggers?) "That is all they are." Asked about her people, she says "They are in Heaven." (Where are you?) "I am in Heaven" (without change of expression). Again, when asked where her people are, says "At home." Then she went willingly back to bed and was quiet. In the afternoon she again went to the door and tried to get out. When questioned, she said "I don't want to be an animal," "Everybody is making an animal of me" (pointing to an animal picture). Then again, while trying the door, repeats in the same affectless manner that she wants to go "to the river," "to the bottom of the river," "to Heaven to see my mother." This last was said in a whining tone, with some tears. She kept turning the knob, tried to get the keys, and struggled impulsively when prevented.

December 23: Though quiet on the whole, when a visitor came yesterday, she ran after this woman saying "I want my generations," and clung to her, and to-day at intervals keeps talking about wanting to see her generations but is often quiet. (Retrospectively she said she wanted to see all her ancestors from the beginning of time.)

[172] *December 27:* Of late often talks affectlessly about wanting to die or wanting to go to Heaven, struggling impulsively to get medicine away from the nurses, asking for poison, trying to drink her own urine, or even the fluid in the bed pan after she had been given an enema, all evidently with suicidal intent.

December 28: Still constant, impulsive and apparently affectless attempts at suicide, tries to get medicine away from nurses, to get the fire extinguisher bottles, a bottle of ink, etc., struggling when prevented.

But when examined quiet, even smiles at a joke. When questioned, denies feeling either worried or depressed. She said she wanted to go home. She gave poor attention to the questions. Later she threw a wet sheet over a patient and laughed (this is rare). Later she slapped another patient. Again she began to talk about wishing to go to the grave. Calls Dr. M. "Uncle John."

December 30: Talks either about wanting to die, or wanting to go to Heaven, or wanting to go to Ireland, all this as usual in an affectless way. Calls Dr. M. "Uncle John." Keeps shouting "Take me to Ireland."

January 9, 1914: Often quiet in bed, again goes to door, talks about wanting to go "to Heaven" or "to Ireland." On the whole, says little.

It seems, then, that the transition was not abrupt, that many traits of the first period remained, but that she was on the whole much quieter, with the exception of some spells when she insisted on going out or killing herself. At such times she showed an affectless, impulsive excitement. Whether there was an element of perplexity then is not clear from the notes. The topics of which she spoke also changed. The idea of wealth was rarely expressed, also the idea of marriage was much in the background, but prominent ideas were those of death, Heaven, killing herself, going to Ireland—all of which she produced in an affectless way. It should be added that she persistently wet and soiled during this, as well as in the first period.

3. Then followed three months of greater inactivity. She lay in bed gazing, moving very little, not even when her meals were brought. She answered but little and consistently wet and soiled. This state lasted from about the middle of February until the beginning of April.

[173] 4. From this stuporous state she emerged during the next four weeks, the awakening being associated with persistent efforts to arouse her. She then was, for six or seven weeks, nearly normal, so far as her mood went, but had a tendency to cling to some of her ideas and was overtalkative. Her memory for the earlier phases of the psychosis was good, as she recalled not only many external events but most of her false ideas. She said, however, that her mind had been a blank for the third stage and she remembered nothing of it. At the end of this time she cleared up entirely and was discharged as "recovered." She continued well for some months, during which she was occasionally examined.

This case gives an excellent example of the relationship of stupor to other manic-depressive reactions. She begins with an absorbed state, showing elements of perplexity and mania. With this there are expansive ideas but, also, statements about losing everything and being in prison, which suggest abandonment of life. Next, with increasing apathy, she begins to speak of death and soon makes impulsive suicidal attempts. Evidently her mind was becoming more and more focused on death and with this there was an appropriate emotional change. She was either apathetic or the affect exhibited itself in pure impulsiveness. Then comes the stupor, when all ideas disappear and mentation is reduced or absent. When the stupor lifts, the original ideas appear not only in memory but occasion a wavering insight. It is appropriate that she recalled all of her psychosis fairly well with the exception of the pure stupor, which she remembered only as a time when her mind was a blank.

Footnotes:

[7] Hoch, August, and Kirby, George H.: "A Clinical Study of Psychoses Characterized by Distressed Perplexity." *Archives of Neurology and Psychiatry*, April, 1919, Vol. I, pp. 415-458.

[8] Hoch, August: "A Study of the Benign Psychoses." *Johns Hopkins Hospital Bulletin*, May, 1915, XXVI, 165.

A book on "the psychology of manic-depressive insanity" will shortly appear by the editor.

[174]

CHAPTER IX
THE PHYSICAL MANIFESTATIONS OF STUPOR

We must now discuss the most difficult of all the aspects of the stupor problem. The subject is so involved and the evidence so inconclusive that observers will probably interpret the phenomena here reported according to their individual preconceptions. What we have to say is therefore published not so much to convince as to stimulate further work. The problem is wider than that of the mere etiology of the stupors we are considering. Their relationship to manic-depressive insanity is so intimate that we must tentatively consider this affectless reaction as belonging to that larger group. A discussion of the basic pathology of manic-depressive insanity is outside the sphere of this book. The author, therefore, thinks it advisable to state somewhat dogmatically his view, as to the etiology of these affective reactions, merely as a starting point for the argument concerning stupors specifically.

It is our view that the manic-depressive psychoses may be, and probably are, determined remotely but fundamentally by an inherent neuropsychic defect, but this physical and constitutional blemish is non-specific. The actual psychosis is determined by [175] functional, that is, psychological factors. A predisposed individual exposed to a certain psychic stress develops a manic-depressive psychosis. Naturally any physical disease reduces the capacity for normal response to mental difficulties; hence physical illness may facilitate the production of a psychosis. But this intercurrent factor is also non-specific.

Such is our view of the etiology of manic-depressive insanity as a whole. When we approach the study of benign stupors, however, difficult problems appear. As will be discussed in a later chapter on the literature, reactions resembling benign stupors occur as a result of toxins, particularly following acute rheumatism. Recently the medical profession has been called on to treat many cases of encephalitis lethargica where similar symptoms are observed. If the resemblance amounted to identity, we would have to admit that a specific toxin may produce a specific mental reaction which we have concluded on other grounds to be psychogenic. As a matter of fact, in two particulars these reactions show relationship to organic delirium. Knauer reports that in post-rheumatic stupors illusions are frequent—an ice bag thought to be a cannon, or a child, etc.—and there are bizarre misinterpretations of the physical condition, such as lying on glass splinters, animals crawling on the body, and so on. Such illusions are, in our experience, not found in stupor, and, on the other hand, are cardinal symptoms of delirium. Further, Knauer reports that even at the height of post-rheumatic stupor, external stimuli make some [176] impression, in that a thoughtful facial expression appears. In deep stupors, such as occurred in our series, this response is not seen. The same phenomenon of "rousing," larval in Knauer's cases, is often well marked in encephalitis lethargica and is, of course, a pathognomonic symptom of delirium. We might therefore think that these conditions are mixtures of two organic tendencies, namely, delirium and coma. It is not impossible that resemblances to benign stupor are due to functional elements appearing in the reduced physical state as additions to the organic symptoms. The prominence of pain might be taken as a likely cause for an instinctive reaction of withdrawal, which would account for the emotional palsy of these conditions on psychogenic grounds. [This argument can be better understood when the chapter on Psychological Explanation of Stupor has been read.] We therefore feel justified in holding that the resemblance of the symptoms of certain plainly organic reactions to those of benign stupor do not necessitate a splitting of these stupors from the manic-depressive group.

When we consider certain bodily manifestations of these typical stupors, however, fresh difficulties are encountered. Unlike depressions, elations and anxieties, certain physical symptoms appear with frequency, even regularity. This would seem to indicate the presence of physical disease. Inasmuch as the most constant of them is fever, the natural conclusion would be that we are dealing with an [177] infection which produces a mental state called stupor. If we were not faced with an obvious relationship to manic-depressive insanity, where such symptoms are usually accidental and intercurrent, we would accept this explanation, but this quandary necessitates further analysis.

Let us first consider the fever. In 35 cases, on whom data of temperature could be found from the records extant, 28 showed fever usually running between 99° and 100°, often up to 101° or slightly over this point. When these cases were analyzed, however, it was found that 27 were typical and 8 atypical, showing pictures resembling those described in the last chapter. Of the latter only one had a rise of temperature, while of the typical group only one was afebrile. Therefore, since out of 27 typical cases 26 had the typical slight fever, we must conclude it to be a highly specific symptom. Of these 28 cases the incidence of the fever was as follows: 8 showed it only on admission; in 7 it was highest on admission but continued at a low rate throughout the rest of the psychosis; in 5 it extended without much variation throughout the psychosis; in 4 it appeared intermittently, while in 2 it was accentuated during periods when the mental symptoms were most pronounced. We see, then, that there is a distinct tendency for the fever to be associated with the onset of the disease.

When we look for other data from which we might discover causes for the fever, we find less than we would like. The records are of observations made, [178] some of them, twenty years ago. Although the mental examinations were careful, the records of the physical symptoms either were not made or were lost in many cases. Consequently our description must be tentative and is published merely to stimulate further research as cases come to the attention of psychiatrists.

One looks, first, for other evidence of infection. Some of the cases were thoroughly examined with modern methods and nothing whatever found. Blood examinations were made in five cases; three of these had rather high temperature with the following blood pictures: Charles O., 103°, leucocytosis of 23,000, with 91.5% polymorphonuclears; Annie G. (Case 1), 103°, leucocytosis of 12,000 to 15,000, and 89% polymorphonuclears; Caroline DeS. (Case 2), 104°, 15,000 leucocytes, no differential made, Widal and diazo reaction negative. These three cases, then, had marked febrile reactions and leucocytosis. It is quite possible that they had infections which were not discovered. Of the other two Rosie K. (Case 11) had a temperature of 100° and 17,500 leucocytes associated with a fetid diarrhea, an unquestioned infection, while Mary C. (Case 7), with a temperature of only 100°, had no rise in number of total white cells but 41% of lymphocytes. This last might be due to an internal secretion or an involuntary nervous system anomaly. The possibility of the three high temperatures with leucocytosis being due to intercurrent infections must be considered. Charles O. had high fever only for ten [179] days during a psychosis of several months. Annie G.'s high fever was of about the same duration. Caroline DeS. had short periods of marked pyrexia in the first and seventh months of her long psychosis. Except for these episodes, these three patients had the typical slight elevation of temperature. Three cases out of thirty-five, in which high fever and leucocytosis appeared episodically, are hardly enough to justify the view that stupors are the result of a specific infection. We must remember, too, that no focal neurological symptoms are ever observed, which makes the possibility of a central nervous system infection highly unlikely.

An alternative view might be that the slight rise of fever is somehow the result of stupor, not the cause of it. The editor consulted Professor Charles R. Stockard, of Cornell Medical College, as to this possibility. The following argument is the result of his suggestions:

What we call a normal temperature is, of course, the result of a balance maintained between heat production and heat loss. Either an increase in the former or a decrease in the latter must produce fever. It is possible that heat production may be increased in many stupors as a result of the muscular rigidity. Some cases showed higher temperature when this was more marked, but this was not sufficiently constant to justify any conclusions being drawn.

Heat loss occurs preponderantly as a result of radiation from the skin and by sweating with conse [180] quent evaporation of the secretion. These processes are functions of the skin and surface circulation. Are they disturbed in our stupors? We find considerable evidence that they are. Flushing or dermatographia occurred in six cases, cold or blue extremities in four cases, greasy skin in four, marked sweating in three, the hair fell out in two cases, while the skin was pathologically dry in one case, in fact there were few patients who showed normal skin function. Circulatory anomalies were also observed. The pulse was very rapid in eleven cases, weak or irregular in two, and slow in one case. All these symptoms are expressions of imbalance in the involuntary nervous system, further evidence of which is found in the rapid respiration of six cases and the shallow breathing of one patient. These pulse and respiration findings are the more striking in that individuals in stupor are, by the very nature of their disease, free from emotional excitement.

This imbalance could result from a poverty of circulating adrenalin which is necessary for the activation of the sympathetic nerves. A cause for low suprarenal function is to be found in the apathy of the stupor case. As Cannon and his associates have so conclusively demonstrated, any emotion which was open to investigation resulted in an increase of adrenalin output. As our emotions are constantly operating during the day — and often enough during sleep as well in connection with dreams — we must presume that emotional stimulus is a normal excitant [181] for the production of adrenalin. It is therefore inconceivable that the blood could receive its normal supply of adrenalin with an apathy of the degree seen in stupor unless some purely hypothetically substitutive excitant were found.

We may therefore tentatively assume that the fever which marks the onset and frequently the course of these benign stupors is the result of a failure of the heat loss function, this being due to an imbalance in the involuntary nervous system that is occasioned, in turn, by insufficient circulating adrenalin, and the final cause for the poor suprarenal function is to be traced to the most consistent symptom of the stupor, namely, apathy. This hypothesis is welcome, not only because it would account adequately for the fever, but it also tends to accentuate the relationship with other forms of manic-depressive insanity, all of which are marked fundamentally by a pathological emotion. Naturally enough, one turns to the records again to see if the blood-pressure of these patients was low, as would be expected with a poor adrenalin supply. Unfortunately record was made of the blood-pressure in only two cases, in both of which the reading was 110 m.m. Two such isolated observations mean, of course, nothing whatever. It is possible that the drooling which so many stupor cases show is not merely the result of the failure of the swallowing reflex, but represents as well a compensation for anhydrosis by excessive salivary secretion.

Another symptom suggestive of involuntary ner [182] vous system or endocrine disorder is the highly frequent suppression of the menstrual function. At times this may occur as a sequel to mental shock, as it did in the case of Celia H. (Case 19), who was menstruating when, frightened by the suicidal attempt of her brother, the flow ceased abruptly. That purely psychic factors can produce marked changes in such functions has been demonstrated by Forel and other hypnotists time and again; presumably the effect is produced by way of alteration in the endocrine or involuntary nervous system influence. In such cases, however, we can trace the menstrual suppression directly to an emotional cause. On the other hand, most women in stupor fail to menstruate during the bulk of the psychosis at a time when we believe emotions to be absent or greatly reduced in their intensity. The recent work of Papanicolaou and Stockard [9] offers a simple explanation for this phenomenon. They have shown that in the guinea pig the œstrous cycle can be delayed by starvation, while in weaker animals a period may be suppressed completely. When one considers that even with the greatest care the nutrition of tube-fed patients is bound to be poor, it would be only natural to suppose that this malnutrition would cause such a disturbance in the œstrous cycle and was evidenced objectively by a failure to menstru [183] ate. Even in patients who are not tube-fed, under-nutrition is to be expected and, as a matter of fact, is usually observed. The work of Pawlow and Cannon has shown how essential psychic stimulus is for gastric digestion. Any condition of apathy would therefore tend to retard digestion and indirectly affect nutrition.

Finally, under the heading of Physical Manifestations of Stupor, we must consider epileptoid attacks, of which there was a history in two of our cases, both of which have already been described in the first chapter of this book. Anna G. (Case 1), in her second attack, was treated at another hospital, and from the account which they sent it appears that the stupor was immediately preceded by a seizure in which the whole body jerked. This is, of course, rather thin evidence of the existence of a definite convulsion, but in the case of Mary F. (Case 3) we have a fuller description. During the two days when the stupor was incubating, she had repeated seizures of the following nature. She sometimes said that prior to the attacks it became dark before her eyes and that her face felt funny or that she had a pain in the stomach which worked toward her right shoulder. The attack would begin when sitting in a chair, with the closing of her eyes, clenching her fists and pounding the side of the chair. She would then get stiff and slide on to the floor, where she would thrash her arms and legs about and move her head to and fro. The warning of the pain working from the stomach to the right shoulder is highly [184] suggestive of an epileptic aura, although the other symptoms mentioned so far could have been considered hysterical or poorly described epileptic phenomena. The rest of the description indicates an epileptic seizure more strongly. She frothed at the mouth and once wet herself during an attack. They lasted only for a few minutes and she would breathe heavily after them. At the end of one attack she wiped the froth from her mouth with her handkerchief and gave it to her aunt, saying, "Burn that, it is poison." This is perhaps a little less like epilepsy. It is plainly impossible for us to say with any positiveness that either these were or were not genuine convulsions, but it is nevertheless important to record them, because such phenomena are observed fairly frequently in dementia præcox cases but are practically unknown in manic-depressive insanity. This, then, would be another example of the resemblance to dementia præcox in these stupors which are unquestionably benign. [10]

[185] We see, then, in reviewing all the physical manifestations of the benign stupors, that none occurred which cannot be explained as secondary to the mental changes, and therefore, until such time as physical symptoms are reported which cannot be so explained, we see no reason for changing our view that the benign stupor is to be regarded as one of the manic-depressive reactions.

Footnotes:

[9] Papanicolaou, G. N., and Stockard, C. R., "Effect of Underfeeding on Ovulation and the Œstrous Rhythm in Guinea-pigs." *Proceedings of the Society of Experimental Biology and Medicine*, Vol. XVII, No. 7, Apr. 21, 1920.

[10] As a matter of fact, if the views of Clark and MacCurdy [B] be accepted, some reason for these epileptic-like attacks may be imagined. According to them, epilepsy is a disease characterized by a lack of the natural instinctive interest in the environment which is expressed chronically in the deterioration, and episodically in the

attacks, the most consistent feature of which is loss of consciousness. Now, in stupor we have an analogous reaction where, although consciousness is not disturbed in the sense in which it is in epilepsy, it is nevertheless considerably affected, inasmuch as contact with the environment is practically non-existent. The coincident thinking disorder is quite similar, both in epileptic dementia and the torpor following seizures and in these benign stupors. MacCurdy has suggested tentatively that the epileptic convulsion may be secondary to a very sudden loss of consciousness which removes a normal inhibition on the muscles, liberating the muscular contractions which constitute the convulsion. If this view were correct, it would not be hard to imagine that during the onset of these stupors the tendency to part company with the environment, which ordinarily comes on slowly, might occur with epileptic suddenness and hence liberate convulsive movements. This is, however, a pure speculation but not fruitless if it serves to draw attention to the analogies existing between the stupor reaction and some of the mental symptoms of epilepsy. These analogies are strong; aside from the obvious clinical differences, the stupor and epileptic reactions are dynamically unlike in that they are the product of different temperaments and precipitated by different situations.

[B] Clark, L. Pierce. "Is Essential Epilepsy a Life Reaction Disorder?" *Am. Jour. of the Medical Sciences*, November, 1910, Vol. CLVIII, No. 5, p. 703. This paper gives a summary of Dr. Clark's theories.

MacCurdy, John T., "A Clinical Study of Epileptic Deterioration." *Psychiatric Bulletin*, April, 1916.

[186]

CHAPTER X
PSYCHOLOGICAL EXPLANATION OF THE STUPOR REACTION

In the previous chapter mention has been made of our view that manic-depressive insanity is a disease fundamentally based on some constitutional defect, presumably physical, but that its symptoms are determined by psychological mechanisms. In accordance with this hypothesis we seek, when studying the different forms of insanity presented in this group, to differentiate between the different types of mental mechanisms observed, and by this analysis to account for the manifestations of the disease on purely psychological lines. If benign stupors belong to this group, then we should be able to find some specific psychology for this type of reaction.

All speech and all conduct, except simple reflex behavior, are presumably determined by ideas. When an individual is not aware of the purpose governing his action, we assume, in psychological study, that an unconscious motive is present, so that in either case the first step in psychological understanding of any normal or abnormal condition is to discover, if possible, what the ideas are that lead to the actions [187] or utterances observed. In the case of stupors the situation is fairly simple, in that the ideational content is extremely limited. As has been seen, it is confined to death and rebirth fancies, other ideas being correlated with secondary symptoms, such as belong to mechanisms of other manic-depressive psychoses. It is not necessary to repeat the catalogue of the typical stupor ideas, as they have been given in an earlier chapter. Our task is now to consider the significance of these death and rebirth delusions and their meaning for the stupor reaction.

Thoughts concerned with future and new activities require energy for their completion in action and are therefore naturally accompanied by a sense of effort which gives pleasure to an active mind. When the sum of energy is reduced, one observes a reverse tendency called "regression." It is easier to go back over the way we know than to go forward, so the weakened individual tends to direct his attention to earlier actions or situations. To meet a new experience one must think logically and keep his attention on things as they are, rather than imagine things as one would like to have them.

Progressive thinking is therefore adaptive, while regressive thinking is fantastic in type, as well as concerned with the past—a past which in fancy takes on the luster of the Golden Age. Sanity and insanity are, roughly speaking, states where progressive or regressive thinking rule. The essence of a functional psychosis is a flight from reality to a retreat of easeful unreality.

[188]

Carried to the extreme, regression leads one in type of thinking and in ideas back to childhood and earliest infancy. The final goal is a state of mental vacuity such as probably characterizes the infant at the time of birth and during the first days of extra-uterine life. In this state what interest there is, is directed entirely to the physical comfort of the individual himself, and contact with the environment is so undeveloped that efforts to obtain from it the primitive wants of warmth and nutrition are confined to vague instinctive cries. Evolution to true contact with the world around implies effort, the exercise of self-control, and also self-sacrifice, since the child soon learns that some kind of *quid pro quo* must be given. Viewed from the adult standpoint, the emptiness of this early mental state must seem like the Nirvana of death. At least death is the only simple term we can use to represent such a complete loss of our habitual mental functions. When life is difficult, we naturally tend to seek death. Were it not for the powerful instinct of self-preservation, suicide would probably be the universal mode of solving our problems. As it is, we reach a compromise, such as that of sleep, in which contact with reality is temporarily abandoned. In so far as sleep is psychologically determined, it is a regressive phenomenon. It is interesting that the most frequent euphemism or metaphor for death is sleep. Sleep is a normal regression. It does not always give the unstable individual sufficient relaxation from the demands of adaptation and so pathological regressions [189] take place, one of which we believe stupor to be. It is important to note that objectively the resemblance between sleep and stupor is striking. So far as mental activity in either state can be discovered by the observer, either the sleeper or the patient in stupor might be dead. Briefly stated, then, our hypothesis of the psychological determination of stupor is that the abnormal individual turns to it as a release from mental anguish, just as the normal human being seeks relief in his bed from physical and mental fatigue. When this desire for refuge takes the shape of a formulated idea, there are delusions of death.

The problem of sleep is, of course, bound up with the physiology of rest, and as recuperation, in a physical sense, necessitates temporary cessation of function, so in the mental sphere we see that relaxation is necessary if our mental operations are to be carried on with continued success. This is probably the teleological meaning of sleep in its psychological aspects, for in it we abandon diurnal adaptive thinking and retire to a world of fancy, very often solving our problems by "sleeping over them." The innate desire for rest and a fresh start is almost as fundamental a human craving as is the tendency to seek release in death. In fact the two are closely associated both in literature and in daily speech, for in many phases we correlate death with new life. If one is to visualize or incorporate the conception of new life in one term, rebirth is the only one which will do it, just as death is the only [190] word which epitomizes the idea of complete cessation of effort. Not unnaturally, therefore, we find in the mythology of our race, in our dreams and in the speech of our insane patients, a frequent correlation of these two ideas, whether it comes in the crude imagery of physical rebirth or projected in fantasies of destruction and rebuilding of the world. Many of our psychotic patients achieve in fancy that for which the Persian poet yearned:

> "Ah Love! could you and I with Him conspire
> To grasp this Sorry Scheme of Things entire,
> Would we not shatter it to bits—and then
> Re-mold it nearer to the Heart's Desire!"

A vision of a new world is a content occurring not infrequently in manic states, but before the universe can be remolded it must be destroyed. Before the individual can enjoy new life, a new birth, he must die, and stupor often marks this death phase of a dominant rebirth fantasy. In this connection it was not without significance to note that stupors almost universally recover by way of attenuation of the stupor symptoms, or in a hypomanic phase where there seems to be an abnormal supply of energy. Antæus-like, they rise with fresh vigor from the Earth. They do not pass into depressions or anxieties.

Rebirth fancies unquestionably, then, contain constructive and progressive elements, but, as has been stated above, any thinking which implies a lapse of contact with the environment is, in so far [191] as that lapse is concerned, regressive, and in consequence rebirth fancies, as dramatized by the stupor patients, are regressive, just as are the delusions of death itself.

It is obvious that an acceptance of death implies rather thorough mental disintegration. Before that takes place there may be some mental conflict. The instinct of self-preservation may prevent the individual from welcoming the notion of dissolution, so that this latter idea, though insistent, is not accepted but reacted to with anxiety; hence we often meet with onsets of stupor characterized by emotional distress. It has already been suggested that death may foreshadow another existence. Often in the psychoses we meet with the idea of eternal union in death with some loved one whom the vicissitudes and restrictions of this life prevent from becoming an earthly partner. This fancy is frequently the basis of elation. Similarly, new life in a religious sense as expressed in the delusion of translation to Heaven, is a common occasion for ecstasy. These formulations of the death idea may occur as tentative solutions of the patient's problems leading to temporary manic episodes while the psychosis is incubating. It seems that stupor as such appears only when death and nullity are accepted.

The above are more or less a priori reasons for regarding the stupor as a regressive reaction. We must now consider the clinical evidence to support this view. In the first place, we always find that stupor occurs in an individual who is unhappy and [192] who has found no other solution than regression for the predicament in which he is. There is nothing specific in the cause of this unhappiness. At times the factors producing it are mainly environmental; at others, the problem is essentially of the patient's own making. Of course almost any type of functional psychosis may emerge from such a state of dissatisfaction, but it is important to note that unlike manic states, for instance, stupors invariably develop from a situation of unhappiness. Quite frequently the choice of the stupor regression is determined by some definitely environmental event which suggests death. This often comes as the actual death of the patient's father (in the case of a woman) or employer, events which inflate the already existing, although perhaps unconscious, desire for mutual death. Again, the precipitating factor may be a situation which adds still another problem and makes the burden of adaptation intolerable, forcing on him the desire for death. In these cases the actual psychosis is sometimes ushered in dramatically with a vision of some dead person (often a woman's father) who beckons, or there are dream-like experiences of burial, drowning, and so on.

A few cases taken at random from our material exemplify these features of the unhappiness in which the psychosis appears as a solution with its development of the death fancy.

Alice R., at the age of 25, was much troubled by worrying over her financial difficulties and the [193] shame of an illegitimate child. Retrospectively she stated, "I was so disgusted I went to bed—I just gave up hope." Shortly before admission she said she was lost and damned, and to the nurse in the Observation Pavilion she pleaded, "Don't let me murder myself and the baby."

Caroline DeS. (Case 2) for some time was worried over the engagement of her favorite brother to a Protestant (herself a Catholic) and the threatened change of his religion. At his engagement dinner she had a sudden excitement, crying out, "I hate her—I love you—papa, don't kill me." This excitement lasted for three weeks, during two of which she was observed, when she spoke frequently of being killed and going to Heaven. The conflict was frankly stated in the words, "I love my father but don't want to die." Then for two weeks she had some fever, was tube-fed, muttered about being killed or showed some elation, there being apparently interrupted stuporous, manic and, possibly, anxiety episodes. Finally she settled down to a year of deep stupor.

Laura A. had for three months poor sleep with depression over her failure in study. Another cause for worry was that her father was home and out of work. She reached a point where she did not care what happened but continued working. Ten days before admission she was not feeling well. The next morning she woke up confused and frightened, speedily became dazed, stunned, could not bring anything to her memory. This rather sudden [194] stupor onset was not accompanied by any false ideas, at least none which the family remembered.

Mary C. (Case 7) was an immigrant who felt lonely in the new country. Two weeks before admission her uncle with whom she was living died. She thought she had brought bad luck, complained of weakness and dizziness, then suddenly felt mixed up, her "memory got bad," and she thought she was going to die. Next she was frightened, heard voices, thought there was shooting and a fire. For a short time she was inactive and later began shouting "Fire!" When taken to the Observation Pavilion, she was dazed, uneasy, thought she was on a boat or shut up in a boat which had gone down; all were drowned. Then came a mild stupor.

Maggie H. (Case 14), while pregnant, fancied that her baby would be deformed and that she would die in childbirth. Three weeks before admission this event took place. For five days she worried about not having enough milk, about her husband losing his job (he did lose it) and thought her head was getting queer. On the fifth day she cried, said she was going to die, that there was poison in the food, that her husband was untrue to her. She became mute but continued to attend to her baby. She saw dead bodies lying around, and by the time she was taken to the Observation Pavilion was in a marked stupor.

Turning now to the symptoms of the stupor proper, we note, first, the effects of the loss of energy which regression implies. The inactivity and [195] apathy which these patients show is too obviously evidence of this to require further comment. Another proof of the withdrawal of the libido or interest is found in the thinking disorder. Directed, accurate thinking requires effort, as we all know from the experience of our laborious mistakes when fatigued. So in stupor there is an inability to perform simple arithmetical problems, poor orientation is observed, and so on. Similarly what we remember seems to be that which we associate with the impressions received by an active consciousness. Actual events persist in memory better than those of fancy, in proof of which one thinks at once of the vanishing of dreams on waking, with its reëstablishment of extroverted consciousness. This registration of impressions requires interest and active attention. Without interest there is no attention and no registration. The patient in stupor presents just the memory defect which we would expect. Indifference to his environment leads to a poor memory of external events, while on recovery there may be such a divorce between consciousness of normal and abnormal states that the past delusions are wiped from the record of conscious memory. Withdrawal of energy then produces not only inactivity and apathy but grave defects in intellectual capacity.

The natural flow of interest in regression is to earlier types of ambition and activity. This is betrayed not merely by the thought content dealing with the youth and childhood of the patient, but also is manifested in behavior. Excluding involution [196] melancholia there is probably no psychosis in which the patients exhibit such infantile reactions as in stupor. Except for the stature and obvious age of these patients, one could easily imagine that he was dealing with a spoiled and fractious infant. One thinks at once of the negativism which is so like that of a perverse child and of the unconventional, personal habits to which these patients cling so stubbornly. Masturbation, for instance, is quite frequent, while willful wetting and soiling is still more common. We sometimes meet with childishness, both in vocabulary and mode of expression. In one case there was evidently a delusion of a return to actual childhood, for she kept insisting that she was "in papa's house."

The frequency with which the delusion of mutual death occurs in stupor is another evidence of its regressive psychology. The partner in the spiritual marriage is rarely, if ever, the natural object of adult affection, but rather a parent or other relative to whose memory the patient has unconsciously clung for many years, reawakening in the psychosis an ambition of childhood for an exclusive possession that reaches its fulfillment in this delusion. Closely allied with this is another delusion, that of being actually dead, which the patients sometimes express in action, even when not in words. The anesthesia to pin pricks, the immobility and the refusal to recognize the existence of the world around, in patients who give evidence of some intellectual operations still persisting, are probably all part of a feigned [197] death, with the delusion expressing itself in corpse-like behavior.

Finally we must consider the meaning of the deep stupor where no mentation of any kind can be proven and where none but vegetative functions seem to be operating. This state is either one of organic coma, in which case it marks the appearance of a physical factor not evidenced in the milder stages, or else it is the acme of this regression by withdrawal of interest. As has been stated, back of the period of primitive childish ideas there lies a hypothetical state of mental nothingness. If we accept the principle of regression we find historically an analogue to what is apparently the mental state of deep stupor in the earliest phases of infancy. This view receives justification from the study of the phenomenon of variations in symptoms. Mental faculties at birth are larval, and if such condition be artificially produced mental activity must be potentially present (as it would not be if we were dealing with coma). In Chapter IV phenomena of interruption of stupor symptoms were detailed. One case that was mentioned is now of particular importance as demonstrating that an appropriate stimulus may dispel the vacuity of complete stupor by raising mental functions to a point where delusions are entertained. This patient retrospectively recalled only certain periods of her deepest stupor, occasions when she was visited by her mother. At these times, as she claimed, she thought she was to be electrocuted and told her mother so, adding, "Then it [198] would drop out of my mind again." Otherwise her memory for this state was a complete blank. Here we see a normal stimulus producing not normality but something on the way towards it, that is, a condition less profound than the state out of which the patient was temporarily lifted.

This case exemplifies the principle of levels in the stupor reaction which we have found to be of great value in our study. These levels are correlated with degrees of regression, as a review of the symptoms discussed above may show. In the first place, the dissatisfaction with life, the first phase of regression, leads to the quietness—the inactivity and apathy, which are the most fundamental symptoms of the stupor reaction as a whole. Initiative is lost and with this comes a tendency for the acceptance of other people's ideas. That is the probable basis for the suggestiveness which we concluded was a prominent factor in catalepsy. Indifference and stolidity may exist with those milder degrees of regression which do not conflict with one's critical sense, and hence may be present without any false ideas. The next stage in regression is that where the idea of death appears. Although not accepted placidly by the subject, its non-acceptance is demonstrated by the idea being projected—by its appearance as a belief that the patient will be killed. This notion of death coming from without has again two phases, one with anxiety where normality is so far retained that the patient's instinct of self-preservation produces fear, and a second phase where this in [199] stinct lapses and the patient so far accepts the idea of being killed as to speak of it with indifference. The next step in regression is marked by the spoiled-child conduct, interest being so self-centered as to lead to autoerotic habits and the perverse reactions which we call negativism. When death is accepted but mental function has not ceased, the latter is confined to a dramatization of death in physical symptoms or to such speech and movements as indicate a belief that the patient is dead, under the water, or in some such unreal situation. Finally, when all evidence of mentation in any form is lacking, we see clinically the condition which we know as deep stupor and which we must regard psychologically as the profoundest regression known to psychopathology, a condition almost as close to physiological unconsciousness as that of the epileptic.

Naturally we do not see individual cases in which all these stages appear successively, each sharply defined from its predecessor. To expect this would be as reasonable as to look for a man whose behavior was determined wholly by his most recent experience. Any psychologist knows that every human being behaves in accordance with influences whose history is recent or represents the habit of a lifetime. At any given minute our behavior is not simply determined by the immediate situation, but is the product of many stages in our development. Quite similarly we should not expect in the psychoses to find evidences of regression to a given period of the individual's life appearing exclusively, but [200] rather we should look for reactions at any given time being determined preponderantly by the type of mentation characteristic for a given stage of his development. As a matter of fact, we see in psychoses, particularly in stupor, more sharply defined regressions to different levels than we ever see in normal life.

Our psychological hypothesis would be incomplete and probably unsound if it could not offer as valid explanations for the atypical features in our stupor reactions as for the typical. The unusual features which one meets in the benign stupors are ideas or mood reactions occurring apparently as interruptions to the settled quietude or in more protracted mild mood reactions, such as vague distress, depression or incomplete manic symptoms, which have been described in the chapter on affect. The interruptions are easily explained by the theory of regression. If stupor represents a complete return to the state of nothingness, then the descent to the Nirvana or the re-ascent from it should be characterized by the type of thinking with the appropriate mood which belongs to less primitive stages of development. A review of our material seems to indicate that there is a definite relationship between the type of onset and the character of the succeeding stupor. For instance, in the cases so far quoted in this book, the onsets characterized by mere worry and unhappiness and gradual withdrawal of interest had all of them typical clinical pictures. On the other hand, of those who began with reactions of definite [201] excitement, anxiety or psychotic depression, there were interruptions which looked like miniature manic-depressive psychoses in all but one case. This would lead one to think that these patients retraced their steps on recovery or with every lifting of the stupor process, moved slightly upward on the same path on which they had traveled in the first regression. The case of Charlotte W. (Case 12), which is fully discussed in the chapter on Ideational Content, offers excellent examples of these principles.

The next atypical feature is the phenomenon of reduction or dissociation of affect, the frequency of which is mentioned in Chapter V. As the law of stupor is apathy, normal emotions should be reduced to indifference and no abnormal moods, such as elation, anxiety or depression, should occur. What often happens is that these psychotic affects appear but incompletely, often in dissociated manifestations. This looks like a combination of two psychotic tendencies, the stupor reduction process which inhibits emotional response and the tendency to develop abnormal affects which characterize other manic-depressive psychoses. There is no general psychological law which makes this view unlikely. One cannot be anxious and happy at the same instant, although one can alternate in his feelings; but one can fail to react adequately to a given stimulus when inhibited by general indifference. In fact it is because apathy is, properly speaking, not [202] a mood but an absence of it, that it can be combined with a true affect. It is possible, therefore, to have a combination of stupor and another manic-depressive reaction, while the others cannot combine but only alternate. [11]

Finally we must discuss the psychological meaning of cases, such as those described in Chapter VIII, where we concluded that there were psychoses resembling stupors superficially. It seemed likely that these patients were absorbed in their own thoughts, rather than being in a condition of mental vacuity. It is not difficult to explain the objective resemblance. All evidence of emotion (apart from subjective feeling tone which the subject may or may not report) is an expression of contact with the outer world. There must be externalization of attention to environment before a mood becomes evident. A moment's reflection will show this to be true, for no further proof is needed than the phenomena of dreaming. The attention being given wholly to fantasies, the subject lies motionless, mute and placid, although passing through varied autistic experiences. Only when the dream becomes too vivid, disturbs sleep and re-directs attention to the environment—only then is emotion objectively [203] betrayed. There is an appearance of apathy and mental vacuity which the dreamer can soon declare to be false. He was feeling and thinking intensely. In any condition, therefore, such as that of perplexity or of an absorbed manic state, the patient may be objectively in the same condition as a typical stupor. The histories of the two psychoses differentiate the two reactions which may be indistinguishable at one interview. The keynote of one reaction is *indifference*, while that of absorption is *distraction*, a perversion of attention to an inner, unreal world.

In summary we may recapitulate our hypotheses. Stupor represents, psychologically speaking, the simplest and completest regression. Adaptation to the actual environment being abandoned, attention reverts to earlier interests, giving symptoms of other manic-depressive reactions in the onset or interruptions, and finally dwindles to complete indifference. The disappearance of affective impulse leads to objective apathy and inactivity, while the intellectual functions fail for lack of emotional power to keep them going. The complicated mental machine lies idle for lack of steam or electricity. The typical ideational content and many of the symptoms of stupor are to be explained as expressions of death, for a regression to a Nirvana-like state can be most easily formulated in such a delusion. Other clinical conditions may temporarily and superficially resemble stupor on account of the [204] attention being misdirected and applied to unproductive imaginations. To employ our metaphor again, in these false stupors the current is switched to another, invisible machine but not cut off as in true stupor.

Footnotes:

[11] The reader will note that this view is opposed to that of Kraepelin, who has written largely on so-called "*mixed conditions*" in manic-depressive insanity. We believe that careful clinical studies confirm our opinion and that his classification is based on less thorough observation and analysis. This subject will be discussed at greater length in a forthcoming book on "The Psychology of Morbid and Normal Emotions," by Dr. MacCurdy.

[205]

CHAPTER XI
MALIGNANT STUPORS

As we have seen, the benign stupors are characterized by apathy, inactivity, mutism, a thinking disorder, catalepsy and negativism. All these symptoms are also found in the stupors occurring in dementia præcox. In fact this symptom complex has usually been regarded as occurring only in a malignant setting. There can be no question about the resemblance of benign to dementia præcox stupors. Even such symptoms as poverty and dissociation of affect, usually regarded as pathognomonic of dementia præcox, have been described in the foregoing chapters. Either recovery in our cases was accidental or there is a distinct clinical group with a good prognosis. If the latter be true, the symptoms must follow definite laws; if they did not, we would have to abandon our principles of psychiatric classification. Naturally, then, we seek to find the differences between the cases that recover and those that do not. There is never any difficulty in diagnosis where a stupor appears as an incident in the course of a recognized case of catatonic dementia præcox. We shall therefore consider only such clinical pictures as resemble those described in this book, in that the [206] symptoms on admission to a hospital or shortly after are those of stupor. It should be our ambition to make a positive diagnosis before failure to recover in a reasonable time leads to a conclusion of chronicity.

It is probably safe to assume, on the basis of as large a series as ours, that the symptoms of stupor *per se* imply no bad prognosis. Further, it has been noted that a relatively pure type of reaction is seen, the symptoms appearing with tolerable consistency. In analyzing the histories of dementia præcox patients, therefore, one looks for inconsistencies among, or additions to, the stupor symptoms. We may say at the outset that we have been able to find no case of malignant stupor that showed what we regard as a typical benign stupor reaction, and it is questionable whether partial stupor as we have described it, ever occurs with a bad prognosis. Usually the discrepant symptoms in the dementia præcox cases are sufficiently marked to enable one to make a positive diagnosis quite soon after the case comes under observation.

The law of benign stupor is a limitation of energy, emotion and ideational content. In dementia præcox we have a re-direction of attention and interest to primitive fantastic thoughts and a consequent perversion of energy and emotion. In many malignant stupors one can detect evidence of this second type of reaction in symptoms that are anomalous for stupor. For instance, one meets with frequent silly and inexplicable giggling. Then, too, smiling, [207] tears or outbursts of rage, the occasions for which are not manifest, are much more frequent than in typical stupor. Similarly, delusional ideas (not concerned with death at all) may appear or the patient may indulge in speech that is quite scattered, not merely fragmentary. Two cases may be cited briefly to illustrate these dementia præcox symptoms superadded to those of stupor.

Case 20. — *Winifred O'M.* Age: 19. Single. Admitted to the Psychiatric Institute May 6, 1911.

F. H. The occurrence of other nervous or mental disease in the family was denied.

P. H. The patient seems to have been rather shy and goody-goody in disposition. According to her mother this seclusiveness did not begin to be markedly noticeable until the winter before her psychosis, when there was some trouble about getting work. She had previously been to a business school. Then she held a position as stenographer temporarily. When this job was over she had a number of positions that did not last long and was once idle for two months. In February (three months before admission) her father was out of work, which added to her worry.

Onset of Psychosis: Nine days before admission a young man died in the house where they lived. The next day her mother insisted on the patient and her sister going to the funeral. On coming home the patient complained of being afraid and having a funny feeling. She woke up at 2:30 that night and lit all the gas, for which she could give no explanation. The day following, or a week before admission, she was slow, confused, could not get her clothes together. The next day she was restless and worried, giving a superficial explanation for the latter. She played the piano a great deal. The following day she was fidgety and cried. At 4 p.m. she was put to bed and appeared to fall asleep. At midnight when a priest called she said to him privately that she was all over the world, that she went to the 12th floor of the Metropolitan Building, that she sat down and took the man's money, $7, and came right away. She recognized the priest. [208] Three days before admission she wanted to stay in bed, kept her eyes closed. When spoken to she would smile but did not open her eyes. She did not pass her urine all day. Her mother then gave her some medicine which the doctor had left. The patient immediately had a peculiar attack in which she heaved her breast, drew her head back, clenched her fists and worked her feet. Saliva escaped from the side of her mouth. This attack lasted some three to five minutes.

Her mother then called an ambulance and she was taken to the *Observation Pavilion*. She thought that the ambulance doctor was an uncle, a soldier in the Philippines, of whom she was very fond. There she remained in bed, with all her muscles relaxed, her mouth constantly open, saying nothing and indeed resisting efforts which were made to get her to open her eyes.

Under Observation: She sat or lay down with her eyes closed and usually limp, although occasionally resistive. There was practically no reaction to pin pricks. Sometimes she opened her mouth as if to speak but rarely did so except in a very low tone and after repeated questioning. Her answers were rarely relevant. To the usual orientation questions she gave no answers that would indicate that she knew where she was. Sometimes she said "Jimmy" when asked her name, and replied to another question, "Jimmy big smile on." Once she said, "I don't know myself — what I am talking for — what I am doing." In general her speech seemed to indicate that her thought was directed entirely inward and that she paid no attention whatever to the questions. In most benign cases such a condition is accompanied by perplexity or a dreamy, dazed expression. This the patient had not. On the other hand, she was sometimes definitely scattered. For example, when asked, How do you feel? she replied, "Large all name." Again to the command, Tell me your trouble, her answer was, "I couldn't tell my mother last night and I can't tell her this night and I can't tell my *proud*." She referred in a fragmentary way to being crazy and to having been dead. She admitted hearing voices but may not have understood the question.

A week after admission, when visited by her mother, the latter asked her to kiss her. The patient opened her mouth widely and put out her tongue. This is a type of response which we have never seen in our benign cases.

[209] Two days later repeated questioning made it evident that the patient knew more about her environment than would be expected, judging from her other symptoms. She gave the month correctly knew that she was in a hospital and told of having recently been visited by her father. At the same interview she spoke of masturbation, of wanting to marry her uncle, and of having been in bed with her father. The last she referred to as a "fall." Such frank incest ideas are never found in benign psychosis in our experience. Other dementia præcox ideas appeared quite soon, for within three days, when she was talking slightly more freely, she spoke of having often imagined she was having sexual experiences as a result of the influence of a man who lived upstairs, and that even when sitting with her family at the table she felt sexual sensations.

Her condition then remained essentially the same for some time. Then about six weeks after admission she became somewhat less resistive, was frequently seen sitting up in bed, moving her lips considerably (without speech) and regarding the surroundings with a bright interested expression and occasionally smiles. About this time she began exposing herself and chewing her finger nails.

Four months after admission she was noted as being very resistive and negativistic, allowing saliva to accumulate in her mouth and making no attempt to keep the flies off her. At the same time she would keep in her mouth food that had been put there without chewing it.

Two months later she seemed to laugh occasionally when other patients did so, but at the same time she showed a cataleptic tendency and was quite mute.

Six months after admission she began to feed herself but rather sloppily. When one would speak to her, she would occasionally smile, but if shaken she would weep silently. About this time she began to do a little work in the ward, pushing a floor polisher.

For the next couple of months her condition was about the same. She would stand around the ward, doing a little work if urged, might even dance if forced to. She was consistently mute. She was dirty but often decorated herself. Rarely she was assaultive.

Then ten months after admission she one day suddenly became [210] talkative, distractible and emotional, laughing and crying. There was with this, however, no open elation. Her talk was obscene, at times flighty, at times definitely scattered. All her habits were filthy.

This pseudomanic episode lasted for a couple of months, and then she settled down to a fairly consistent deterioration with indifference, silly laughter, occasional assaultiveness, destructiveness and untidiness.

Nearly two years after admission she had another period of excitement lasting about a couple of months. Shortly after this she began to fail physically, and in November, 1913, two years and five months after her admission, she died of pulmonary tuberculosis.

In summary, then, we see that this patient exhibited symptoms of dementia præcox from the outset of her stupor, with scattering, genital sensations and incest ideas. The stupor symptoms gradually gave way to the typical indifference, negativism, obscenity, filthiness and inexplicable conduct of dementia præcox. At the beginning, however, the condition was superficially similar to that of a benign stupor, it being only on careful observation that other symptoms were noted.

Case 21.—*Rose S.* Age: 23. Admitted to the Psychiatric Institute April 5, 1905.

F. H. The mother was living, the father dead. Otherwise no pertinent information was secured.

P. H. The patient was said always to have been somewhat seclusive, mingling little with other people; this tendency was so strong that she would leave the room when visitors came. She always slept a great deal. It was stated that she was able to do heavy housework quite well, but never learned cooking.

At 16 she hired out as a servant for a year and a half, and then did laundry work. When 18 she had an illegitimate child by a co-worker.

[211] *History of Psychosis:* About a year before admission the patient's sister was burned to death. When the patient heard of this she said that something had come up in her throat. Henceforth she often complained of a lump in her throat, and often bit her nails. Two months before admission she suddenly left the laundry, again spoke of the lump in her throat, and claimed to have seen the dead sister. Two weeks later when the family had an anniversary mass for the sister the patient appeared sad, but the following day laughed, said she had seen her "sister beckoning her to come." She also thought she saw her picture "and Heaven was behind it." She also talked of "dead relatives and friends." A reaction of levity in connection with a sister's death is highly suggestive of a malignant psychosis.

Two weeks before admission her mother found her in a stupor, immovable, with her eyes closed. In 24 hours she woke up, began to sing "Rest for the Weary," prayed, then was stuporous again for six hours. When she came out of this, she said she was "going to die," God had told her so and talked of her own funeral arrangements. She again went into a stupor, in which she was sent to the Observation Pavilion.

At the *Observation Pavilion* she was described as happy, laughing, singing, saying she felt happy, but adding, "I like to be sad too, I am going to Heaven Easter Sunday." She claimed that her sister frequently stood in front of her, and that she knew she wanted her to go with her.

Under Observation: For about three weeks the patient showed a variable stupor. She would lie with a mask-like face inaccessible, cataleptic, drooling saliva, often with her mouth open. When taken up, she was usually perfectly flaccid, but once she let herself slide on the floor after she had stood immobile at the window. Sometimes there was marked resistance to passive motions, especially when attempts were made to open her mouth or eyes, or on one occasion when the examiner tried to open her hand in which she held her handkerchief. Yet when one persisted in urging her to respond there frequently could be elicited more or less marked reactions. Thus repeatedly she could be made to obey some commands, as showing the tongue, etc., even when she would not answer. Once when her eyes were opened, tears rolled down her cheeks—again, she usually reacted to pin pricks by [212] slight flushing, once she said, "Stop! it hurts." Again, she said, "Leave me alone, I want to sleep."

So far the description of this reaction is that of a benign stupor. There were, however, other symptoms. In the first place, she could sometimes be made to open her eyes and write, although she would not speak. In spite of the penmanship being careless, there were no mistakes. This exhibition of an unhabitual and more difficult intellectual effort when the patient was mute is suggestive of an inconsistency. So was her habit of sometimes singing a hymn, "Rest for the Weary," when no other sign of mental life was given. But, more important than these, she could not infrequently be induced to answer questions and at such times she spoke promptly and with natural affective response.

A number of her replies were of the type to be expected in a benign stupor. In the first place, she spoke of her condition as "going off to sleep" and also as "death," "I was dead all day." "I died three times yesterday," or she merely described it by saying "I go off into states when I lie with my mouth open and eyes closed, and cannot speak or open my eyes." When asked how she got into this condition, she said "My sister died and I think it was on my mind." Again she said she became sad at the anniversary mass of the sister and had been sad ever since. On the other hand, she also stated that when she came home from the mass she first was silly and danced. Spontaneously she spoke of having frequently had visions of her dead sister; once she saw her with wings. In explanation of her singing "Rest for the Weary," she said it was the hymn sung at her father's funeral. An anomalous feature had to do with her description of her feelings. She claimed to have no memory of her stupor periods and yet said of them: "I feel peaceful-like," or "I feel awfully happy and sad together," or "I am sad and contented—I like it that way."

A striking symptom was that, when a sensory examination was made during the first few days during one of the periods when she responded well, she showed glove and stocking anesthesia, also anesthesia of neck and left breast.

But in addition to the above statements the patient also began to make others of a definite dementia præcox type. About ten days after admission she said, "What any one says goes right [213] through my brain," or she talked of being hypnotized. "The typewriting machine turned my eyes—three or four girls turned my eyes—they look at me and get their chance, their left eye—turning me into images. I want to be the way I was born—turn my body! look how their bodies are turned before they die," or "Take it if you get it—he got the name out—I was over there to death—himself to death—of, you know—you played out—she is played out." ... This while she snickered between the sentences. As early as four weeks after admission she had begun to giggle or laugh, often in an empty fashion, and a transition from the more constrained stuporous state, with interruptions of laughter, to an indifferent silly, muttering to herself was gradual.

In 1909 she was described as not talking, standing around, showing no interest in anything, muttering. The only response obtained was "I don't know." In December, 1911, she was transferred to another hospital as a case of deteriorated dementia præcox.

To Recapitulate: We have here a young woman who for a year had indefinite mental symptoms and suddenly developed a stupor. This was atypical in that she sang and wrote when otherwise apparently deeply stuporous. When persuaded to talk, her utterances, even as early as ten days after admission, were of a malignant type and with such statements she giggled. This last is apparently a highly important sign. Quite frequently in our cases the first signal of a dementia præcox reaction has been giggling in a setting of what was apparently a typical benign stupor.

As has frequently been stated, symptoms of benign stupor are closely interrelated. Consequently the reaction is, when benign, a consistent one. We do not find free speech with profound apathy and in [214] activity, nor do we expect to meet with unimpaired intellectual functions when other evidences of deep stupor are present. The inconsistency of mental operations which characterize dementia præcox, however—the "splitting" tendency which Bleuler has emphasized in his term "schizophrenia"—is just that added factor which may produce disproportionate developments of the various stupor symptoms in the dementia præcox type of that reaction. Examples of this have been given in the two cases just quoted. The history of the following patient shows this tendency more prominently.

Case 22.—*Nellie H.* Age: 20. Admitted to the Psychiatric Institute June 11, 1907.

F. H. The father had repeated depressions; he died of typhus fever. The mother was living.

P. H. The brother of the patient stated that she was like other girls, and very good at school. At 16 she became quieter, less energetic. She came to America at 17. After arriving here she has seemed low spirited, cranky and faultfinding. She often complained of indefinite stomach trouble and headaches; when at home she often had a cloth around her head. The informant recalled that she said, "I wish I could get sick for a long time and get either cured or die." However, she worked. For one and a half years prior to admission her "crankiness" is said to have become much worse. She complained continually of being tired; quarreled much with her mother; said she did not have enough to eat. It is also stated that she was constantly afraid of losing her job.

History of Psychosis: For six months before admission she said frequently that her boss was giving her hints that he liked her. (She did not know him socially at all.) Six days before admission she came home, saying the boss had told her he had no more work for her. Nevertheless, she went back next day and was again sent home. At home she sat gazing. Next day again [215] wanted to go and see the boss, but was prevented. At times she tried to get out of the window; again sat gazing, repeating to herself "Always be true." She said she was in love with the boss. When the doctor gave her medicine she thought it was poison. Finally she began to be talkative and elated. At the *Observation Pavilion* she became very quiet.

Under Observation: She lay in bed indifferent, not eating, unless spoon-fed, when she would swallow. She soiled herself. She answered no questions as a rule, and only on one occasion, when urged considerably, said in answer to questions that this was a hospital, so that she evidently had more grasp on the nature of her environment than her behavior indicated. To her brother who called on her during the first ten days she said she could not find her lover here (an idea inconsistent with the benign stupor picture).

Then she became more markedly stuporous, drooling saliva, very stiff, often lying with head half raised, gazing stolidly, never answering, soiling. Later, after a month, this was less consistent. She now and then went to the closet, sometimes she smiled, ate some fruit brought to her, spoke a little. Repeatedly when people came she clung to them, wanted to go home, again was seen to weep silently. On another occasion she suddenly threw the dishes on the floor with an angry mood, without there being any obvious provocation. Again she got quite angry when urged to eat her breakfast, and on that occasion pulled out some of her own hair. Usually she had to be fed, was stiff, sitting with closed fists, not reacting as a rule in any other way, wholly inaccessible and has been that way for years. The stupor merged into a catatonic state merely by the development of the inconsistency in her affective reactions.

We see then that inconsistencies among the stupor symptoms themselves and the intrusion of definitely dementia præcox symptoms differentiate the malignant from the benign reactions. As a matter of fact, we find, as a rule, that careful examination of the onset reveals further atypical features, sugges [216] tions or definite evidences of a dementia præcox reaction before the stupor itself appears. One common occurrence is a slow deterioration of character and energy that proceeds for months or years before flagrantly psychotic symptoms appear.

Then when delusions or hallucinations are eventually spoken of by the patient, an appropriate or adequate reaction is lacking. In a benign psychosis false ideas do not appear with an equable mood unless the stupor reaction has already begun.

More important than this, although in benign stupors there may be a reduction or an insufficient affect, it is never inappropriate. This pathognomonic symptom of dementia præcox frequently occurs in the onset to malignant stupors. In fact we often find in reviewing such cases that a plain dementia præcox reaction has been in evidence, that a diagnosis has not been made simply because the stupor picture blotted out this earlier psychosis before an opinion was formed. Frequently these early symptoms are reported in the anamnesis and not actually observed by the physician.

Three cases may be cited as examples of dementia præcox onsets. It will be noted that the ensuing stupors were, like those already quoted, atypical.

Case 23.—*Catherine H.* Age: 21. Admitted to the Psychiatric Institute October 10, 1904.

F. H. The mother's brother had two attacks of delirium tremens. The mother died when the patient was eleven years old; she is said to have been normal. The father was living.

P. H. The patient was always a nervous child, had very bad [217] dreams, but she was smart at school up to ten or eleven, and played with other girls. Then she began to work less well, got thin, more nervous, complained of headaches. It was about that time that her mother died. (The reaction to the death was said not to have been different from that of her sister.) She was kept at home and was quiet.... "You could see something was working on her." She began to menstruate at 14, and it was claimed that she then wakened up a little. It was further stated that she was always "stuck up" about her clothes.

At 16 she went to work in a factory, but her sister thought the work was too much for her, so she was taken home. Thereafter she lived alone with her father, doing his housework, her sister having married about that time. At 17 her hair began to come out excessively, so that she had to cut it, and when it grew again it was gray. She became very sensitive about this, even refused to take positions because she thought people would remark about it.

For two years before admission she evidently was different. Although she did her father's housework well enough, she turned against her sister and refused to speak to her because, she alleged, the sister had not come to help her in her housework. Another pronounced manifestation during that time was her frequent talk about her bowels. She complained of constipation, creepy, crawling sensations in the stomach which she thought was a "tapeworm." She got pamphlets and took patent medicines. She was taken to a physician nine months before admission, who operated on her for piles. While still in the hospital she asked her father to take her home to die (although there was no reason for such a request). Again she said the gauze had been left in the rectum too long and that the rectum was full of wind. Later she said the rectum was closing up. After this, the sister stated, she was extremely nervous if she passed a day without a movement of the bowels. She was quiet henceforth, went out less and said little, claiming it was better for her head if she said little. She often sat, head in hand, in the hall. All through the summer she frequently remarked, "I am a good girl." Four months before admission during a period of five weeks she would let her bowels move when standing up. This was relieved by enemas. The father states that she was cranky to him, that sometimes when [218] he merely asked a question she would say, "You hurt my feelings," and once, "You break my heart." Occasionally she seemed to worry about the money spent for her on doctors and medicine.

About two months before admission she said everybody was looking at her. Ten days before admission she said, "I have been sick all this time and thought I was going to die. Now I think Tom (her brother) is going to die." She became fearful of being left alone. Finally she went to the priest, who told her to go home. Then she prayed, leaving the candles burning in the room. That night she was found kneeling before a church in her nightgown. Again she threw a lot of articles into the yard, saying a curse had been put on her by her father, and she did not wish to give him anything. When she was taken to the Observation Pavilion she said, "I am a good girl — my mother is dead — it is all my father's fault."

At the *Observation Pavilion* she put her arm under a hot water faucet "to save the world," prayed and laughed — again sank back and appeared as if asleep. She said, "I hear angels telling me how to pray when I lose my thoughts — sisters and nuns are all around me here, to save and purify the world now and forever, and at the hour of our death."

Under Observation: On admission the patient kept her eyes closed, sang hymns in measured tones, or prayed, or showed a certain ecstasy in her face while her lips quivered and tears ran down her cheeks. On the whole, she answered few questions. When asked how she felt, she said she was happy. (Why do you cry?) "I was crying when I asked God to save souls." (Are you afraid?) "Not now, I have been afraid of everything on Earth ever since my mother died." (What do you mean?) "No one would look at me or talk to me—they said I was a bad girl, but I was pure." Again she said, "They laughed about me, talked about me—and they drew up a play about me—Devil's Island." Or she spoke about having had stomach trouble, bowel trouble, teeth trouble, eye trouble, compound, complicated trouble. (What do you mean?) "Father scolding all the time, he sent me to get bug medicine (true). God gives that medicine to the one that started all the trouble—Devil's Island."

She soiled her bed and was asked why she did it. She said "I have been transformed into a baby, the Lord said I was too [219] pure to be a woman—I had to become a baby to save the world." Or when asked her name she called herself "Baby Chadwick of the whole world—divine Irish Catholic World—Amen," or again "I am the Roman Catholic Irish Divine Baby."

Although she was not essentially disoriented she called the place "mid-heaven," or "a holy house, sort of a hospital." She also said, "In two years more there will be a new world and it will be more happy and holy."

The day after entrance the patient, though in part as described, had a spell when she kept her eyes closed and was rigid. Spells like these returned. (About a month after admission she became completely stuporous.) She prayed at times, at other times was constrained, or kept her eyes closed. Her orientation throughout was good. The content of her psychosis, in addition to the praying attitude, had a more or less vague religious coloring. Thus she called the hospital the "House of God." Again, when on one occasion she had jumped at the window guard and was asked "why?" she said "holy communion." Again she said she was "Mary, Virgin Mother." But this religious trend was intermingled with remarkable elements of another sort. Thus when in order to study her knowledge of the events after admission, she was asked what she had done when she was brought into the ward, she said, "I went into the sanctuary where my bowels moved and water passed from me." (Why do you call it sanctuary?) "Because Jesus did the same thing I did."

Possibly vague sexual allusions are also contained in the following: She said one day to the doctor, "Everything went wrong last night, good, pure, true and holy doctor, I led you astray and you were dying last night, may the Almighty God forgive me, I ought to have died, but I fought it out, for, if I had died, my mother's soul would not have been saved in Heaven and from the flames of Hell." Again, "I will not look at you again, good, pure, holy doctor of the world." (Why?) "I am afraid I will lead you astray." And also: "I led James. Peter astray too." It should be added that she sometimes masturbated rather shamelessly.

She said she heard her mother's voice. (What did she say?) "Something in the sky for me, angels call for me." (What do the angels say?) "The name of my good mother in Heaven." Again [220] she said she had heard her mother the night she came here. (What did she say?) "It was like a voice—feed the calf—that means me, I suppose."

Then after a month the stupor became more continuous. She lay totally inactive for the most part, had to be fed, soiled herself, drooled saliva, was at times cataleptic, often rigid. Her limbs became cyanotic. A few times tears were seen. On other occasions she whispered "peace," or "peace for hazing," or "pray—peace," or "I like to be good." Usually no responses could be obtained.

After some months she was at times seen laughing. This gradually passed into a state of total disinterestedness and inaccessibility. She could finally be made to polish the floor in an automatic fashion, but never spoke, and five years after admission she was transferred to another hospital, where she died (eleven years after admission to the ward of the Institute) without any change in her mental condition having taken place.

Case 24.—*Adele M.* Age: 22. Admitted to the Psychiatric Institute November 11, 1904.

P. H. The father stated that the patient was always "cranky," had outbursts of temper, even when a small child and was quarrelsome; also said that she was "seclusive," had few friends, was averse to meeting people, never had a beau. She was taken out of school at 14 because she was not promoted on two successive occasions from the same class. Then she was put to work, but she was usually discharged for incompetency.

Onset of Psychosis: Three years before admission it was noted that she laughed occasionally without cause. She was idle. This laughing, and also crying, was sometimes more frequent, again less noticeable.

Six months before admission she began to say she wanted to leave home, but made no move to do so. Then she began to speak of bad odors, made some remarks about the neighbors talking about her—saying she should kill herself; again she said the family would be brought to death, or the mother was falling to pieces, the father looked sick. She also said her head was swelling and was getting thick. Finally she wanted to hire a furnished room and kill herself and asked if 75 cents which she had was enough to do it with.

[221] Two weeks before admission she left home, wandered about all night, was picked up by the Salvation Army, and returned to her home. She said she wanted to die.

At the *Observation Pavilion* she stated that her mother was falling to pieces and her father sick. She also said she wanted to die.

Under Observation: The patient was at first petulant, saying "I don't want to stay here," turning her face away from the doctor, generally uninterested. Though it could be established that she was quite oriented, often her answers were "I don't know," or she did not answer. But she was also seen crying at times, and she was apt to bite her finger nails. She had to be tube-fed. Gradually these tendencies increased so that she lay in her bed with head covered, saying in a peevish tone, when spoken to, "Oh, let me alone." And for years she was mute, lying with her head covered, tube-fed. When reëxamined in 1914 (ten years later), she was found lying in bed with an empty smile. There was paper stuffed in her ears. When approached, she turned her head away and would not talk.

Case 25.—*Catherine W.* Age: 42. Admitted to the Psychiatric Institute November 11, 1904.

F. H. The father died at 75, the mother at 44. Two sisters died of tuberculosis. A brother wanted to marry but was opposed by the father; he set fire to the house of the girl and then drowned himself.

P. H. The patient came to this country when 20, and worked for some years as a servant. Then she married after a short acquaintance. The husband, according to his own statement, drank, and there was friction from the first. She left him a few weeks after marriage, and a few months later he went to Ireland; she also went some time later but did not go to see him. Then they lived together again. They had four children, but had had no intercourse for nine years.

Development of Psychosis: Eight years before admission the patient became nervous, slept badly, but got better. It was claimed that for six years she had been quieter and more sullen than before. Three years before admission the patient had to take a place as janitress, since she needed the money. From the first she had trouble with the tenants and accused everybody of [222] being in league against her. Some six or eight weeks after she had taken the position, she developed what was called typhoid fever, and some time later the daughter came down with the same disease. After the typhoid she was more antagonistic towards her husband, accused him of infidelity, repeatedly locked him out of the house, but continued to do her housework. About six months after this illness she left her home, but returned in a week. She had vague ideas thereafter that the priests were saying things against the family, and she often quarreled with the tenants. For a year she had done no work but sat about. Ten days before admission she stopped eating.

Under Observation: The patient was mute, stolid, gazing straight ahead, sometimes cataleptic. She had to be tube-fed, was usually very resistive to any passive motions; quite often she retained her urine, but she did not hold her saliva. Yet there was some quick responses at least in the beginning. At such times it was found that she was oriented, but nothing could ever be obtained about her feelings, etc., except that she once said, when asked whether she was worried, that she "felt weak," had "nothing to worry about." Occasionally she was seen to cry silently; at times she would breathe faster when questioned, or flush; once she took hold of the doctor's hand when he questioned her, and cried, but made no reply. On another occasion she was affectionate to her son, kissed him, although she paid no attention to her daughter who accompanied the son. Later she said to the nurses, "He is the best son that ever lived." But more and more she became disinterested, totally inaccessible, resistive, had to be tube-fed. In this condition she remained for five and a half years. At the end of that time she died of tubercular pneumonia.

[223]

CHAPTER XII
DIAGNOSIS OF STUPOR

In any functional psychosis an offhand diagnosis is dangerous. When one deals with such a condition as stupor, however, the problem is exacting, for, although "stupor" may be seen at a glance, what is seen is really only a symptom or a few symptoms. "Stupor," then, is more of a descriptive than a diagnostic term. The real problem is to determine the psychiatric group into which the case should be placed. This is a difficult task, for the differential diagnosis rests on the observation and utilization of minute and unobtrusive details. A correct interpretation can be only reached by obtaining a complete history of the onset and observing the behavior and speech of the patient for a long period, usually of weeks, sometimes of months. With these precautionary words in mind, it may be well to summarize briefly the diagnostic problems in connection with benign stupor.

In the first place one naturally considers the differentiation from conditions of organic stupor or coma. Since psychotic stupors never develop without some signs of mental abnormality, the history is usually a sufficient basis for final judgment. [224] In case no anamnesis is obtainable the functional nature of the trouble may be recognized by the absence of those physical signs which characterize the organic stupors. One sees no violent changes in respiration, pulse or blood-pressure, such as are present in the intoxication comas of diabetes or nephritis. There is no characteristic odor to the breath, and the urine is relatively normal. The unconsciousness of trauma or apoplexy is accompanied by focal neurological signs. Even in aerial concussion (so frequently seen in the war) where no one part of the brain is demonstrably affected more than another, there are neurological evidences of what one might call "physiological" unconsciousness. The eyes roll independently, the pupils fail to react to light. On the other hand, there are definite symptoms characteristic of the functional state. Mental activity is evidenced by a muscular resistiveness or retention of urine. Even in states of complete relaxation the eyes move in unison, the pupils react to light, and almost universally the corneal reflex is present. The patient appears in a deep sleep rather than actually unconscious.

The post-epileptic sleep may resemble a stupor strongly. But this condition is temporary and the situation and appearance of the patient betrays the fact that he has just had a convulsion. Rarely, protracted stuporous states occur in epilepsy which closely resemble the conditions described in this book. In fact it is probable the true stupors may [225] occur in epilepsy just as in dementia præcox or manic-depressive insanity.

There is usually little difficulty in the discrimination of hysterical stupor. Occasionally it shows, superficially, a similarity to the manic-depressive type. Fundamentally, there is a wide divergence between the two processes, in that in the hysterical form a dissociation of consciousness takes place, the patient living in a reminiscent, imaginary or artificially suggested environment, while in a true stupor there is a withdrawal of interest as a whole and a consequent diffuse reduction of all mental processes. This difference is sooner or later manifested by the appearance in the hysteric of conduct or speech embodying definite and elaborated ideas.

As has been stated fully in the last chapter (to which the reader is referred), the stupor of dementia præcox is to be differentiated from that of manic-depressive insanity by the inconsistency of the symptoms in the former and the appearance of dementia præcox features during the stupor, such as inappropriate affect, giggling, or scattering. Further, the nature of the disorder is usually manifest before the onset of the stupor as such.

Sometimes very puzzling cases occur in more advanced years when it is difficult to say whether one is dealing with involution melancholia or stupor. Such patients show inactivity, considerable apathy and wetting and soiling, and with these a whining hypochondria, negativism, and often a rather mawkish sentimental death content without the dramatic [226] anxiety which usually characterizes the involution state. In these cases the diagnosis is bound to be a matter of taste. In our opinion it is probably better to regard these as clinically impure types. They may be looked on as, fundamentally, involution melancholias (the course of the disease is protracted, if not chronic) in whom the regressive process characteristic of stupor is present as well as that of involution.

Great difficulties are also met with in the manic-depressive group proper. So often a stupor begins with the same indefinite kind of upset as does another psychosis that the development may furnish no clew. Any condition where there is inactivity, scanty verbal productivity and poor intellectual performance resembles stupor. This triad of symptoms occurs in retarded depressions, in absorbed manic states and in perplexities. Negativism and catalepsy are never well developed except in stupor. So if these symptoms be present the diagnosis is simplified. But they are often absent from a typical stupor. Let us consider these three groups separately.

The most important difference between stupor and depression lies in the affect. Although inactive and sometimes appearing dull the depressive individual is not apathetic but is suffering acutely. He feels himself wicked, paralyzed by hopelessness, and finds proof of his damnation in the apparent change of the world to his eyes and in the slowness of his mind. But he is acutely aware of these torments. [227] The stupor patient, on the other hand, does not care. He is neither sad nor happy nor anxious. This contrast is revealed not only by the patients' utterances but by their expressions. The stuporous face is empty, that of the other lined with melancholy. The intellectual defect, too, is different. In retarded depression the patient is morbidly aware of difficulty and slowness, but on urging often performs tests surprisingly well. In the stupor, however, one is faced with an unquestionable defect, a sheer intellectual incapacity.

In Chapter VIII the differential diagnosis between perplexity and stupor has already been touched upon. Here again the affect is a point of contrast. The patient has not too little emotion but too much. The feeling of intangible, puzzling ideas and of an insecure environment causes the subject distress, of which complaint is made and which can be witnessed in the furrowed brow and constrained expression. There is also, as we have seen, a rich ideational content in these cases, if one can get at it. The mind is not a blank, as in the stupor, or concerned only with delusions of death.

Finally, there are the absorbed manic states. These are the most difficult, inasmuch as the patient is often so withdrawn and so introverted that at any given interview there may be no objective evidence of mood or ideas. Here the development of the psychosis is often an aid to diagnosis. The patient passes through phases of hypomania to great exultation, the flight becomes less intelligible, with this [228] the activity diminishes until finally expression in any form disappears. If this sequence has not been observed, continued observation tells the tale. The patient still has his ideas and may be seen smiling contentedly over them (not vacuously as does the schizophrenic) or he may break into some prank or begin to sing. Any protracted familiarity with the case leads to a conviction that the patient's mind is not a blank, but that his attention is merely directed exclusively inward. Then, too, when his ideas are discovered, it is found that they are not exclusively occupied with the topic of death.

[229]

CHAPTER XIII
TREATMENT OF STUPOR

In dealing with cases of benign stupor the first duty of physician and nurse is naturally the physical hygiene of the patient. More is needed to be done in the bodily care of these persons than for most of the inmates of our hospitals for the insane. It is perhaps no exaggeration to claim that a deeply stuporous patient needs as much attention as a suckling babe. In the first place, the patient must be fed. It is important for mental recovery that the individual in stupor should be stimulated to effort as much as possible. Consequently there is an economy of time in the long run in taking pains to get the patient to feed himself in so far as that is possible. He should be led to the table and assisted in handling his own spoon and cup. If this is not practicable, he should then be spoon-fed, and if this in turn is found to be out of the question, tube-feeding should be resorted to. But this last should never be looked on as a permanent necessity, but only as a method of maintaining the patient's health until such time as he may be capable of independent taking of nourishment. In exactly the same way it is of prime importance to get the patient to attend [230] to the natural habits of excretion. He should be led to the toilet or to a chair commode, and efforts to this end should be persistent, just as are those of a good child's nurse who has the ambition of making her charge develop normal habits. Naturally those who retain urine and feces should be watched to see that this retention does not last long enough to menace health. The physical aspects of treatment are exhausted with consideration for cleanliness. On account of the stupor patients' inactivity and frequent tendency to wetting and soiling, this is a particularly important consideration. It goes without saying that the perineal region should be kept scrupulously clean. If any infections are to be avoided, eyes, nose and mouth should also be cleansed frequently. A patient who is so indifferent as to keep the eyelids open for such a long time that the sclera dry and ulcerate is also apt to let flies settle and produce serious ophthalmic disease.

Less obvious and more important are the measures undertaken for the mental hygiene of the case. On account of the tendency present in so many patients for sudden action while in the midst of an apparently deep and permanent inactivity, it is necessary that these cases be not isolated but remain under constant observation. This is particularly true of those who have demonstrated impulsive suicidal explosions.

Not only on the basis of the psychological theory of the stupor process, but from the observed phe [231] nomena of recovery, we gather that mental stimulation is of first importance if an amelioration of the condition is to be attempted. If the stupor reaction be a regression, which is essentially a withdrawal of interest and energy rather than a fixation on a false object, then excitement is desirable and interest must be reawakened. The withdrawal is temporary (inasmuch as the psychosis is benign), but just as a normal person wakes more readily on a clear sunshiny day than when it rains, so the more cheering the environment the more rapid the recovery.

Consequently, although trying to those in charge, persistent attention should be given the patient. Feeding and hygienic measures probably have considerable value in this work. As soon as it is at all possible the patients should be got out of bed and dressed. When up, efforts should be directed towards making them do something, even if it be something as simple as pushing a floor polisher. On account of their lack of enthusiasm the stupor cases are often omitted from the list of those given occupation and amusement. Even if they go through the motions of work or play with no sign of interest, such exercise should not be allowed to lapse. Then, too, the environment should be changed when practicable. A patient may improve on being moved to another building.

Perhaps the most potent stimulus that we have observed is that of family visits. In most manic-depressive psychoses visits of relations have a [232] bad effect. The patients become excited, treat the visitors rudely, perhaps even assault them, and all their symptoms are aggravated. But the stupor needs excitement, and an habitual emotional interest is more apt to arouse him than an artificial one. In another point the situation differs. As a rule manic-depressive patients have delusional ideas or attitudes in connection with their nearest of kin, so that contact with these stirs up the trouble. The stupor regression going beneath the level of such attachments leaves family relationships relatively undisturbed. Hence, while the visit of a husband is likely to produce nothing but vituperation or blows from a manic wife, the stuporous woman may greet him affectionately and regain thereby some contact with the world.

So many cases begin recovery in this manner that it cannot be mere chance. One patient's improvement, for instance, dated definitely from the day a nurse persuaded her to write a letter home. It is striking, too, how quickly a patient, while somewhat dull and slow, will brighten up when allowed to return home. A similar improvement under these circumstances is often seen in partially recovered cases of involution melancholia, in whom a psychological regression similar to that of stupor takes place. Such experiences make one wonder whether perhaps these alone of all our insane patients would not recover more quickly at home than in hospitals, provided nursing care could be given them.

This is a mere suggestion. Before treatment can [233] be rational the nature of any disease process must be known, and we do not pretend to have done more as yet than outline the probable mental pathology of the benign stupors. The next step is to put theory into practice and experiment widely with various means to see if by appropriate stimulation the average duration of these psychoses cannot be reduced. It is largely with the hope of inducing other psychiatrists to carry on such work that this book is written. There is no other manic-depressive psychosis which, theoretically, offers such hope of simple psychological measures being of therapeutic value.

[234]

CHAPTER XIV
SUMMARY OF THE STUPOR REACTION

Having discussed in detail the various symptoms and theoretic aspects of the benign stupors, it may be well to have these observations and speculations summarized.

It being established that stupors occur as a temporary form of insanity [12] psychiatry is faced at once with the problem of describing these conditions accurately in order to ascertain their nosological position. To this end we first examined typical cases of deep stupor and found that the clinical picture is made up of the following symptoms: In the foreground stands *poverty of affect*. The patients are almost unbelievably apathetic, giving no evidence by speech or action of interest in themselves or their environment, unmoved even by painful stimuli. Their faces are wooden masks; their voices as colorless when words are uttered. In some cases sudden mood reactions break through at rare intervals. The second cardinal symptom is *inactivity*. As a rule there is a complete cessation of both spontaneous and reactive movements and speech. So profound may this [235] inhibition be that swallowing and blinking of the eyes are often absent. The trouble is not a paralysis, however, for reflexes without psychic components are unaffected. Possibly related to the inactivity is the preservation of artificial positions which is called *catalepsy*, a fairly frequent phenomenon. A tendency opposite to the inactivity is seen in *negativism*. This perversity is present in all gradations from outbursts of anger with blows and vituperation to sullen, or even emotionless, muscular rigidity. This last occurs most often when the patient is approached but may be seen when observations are made at a distance. Frequently *wetting* and *soiling* are due to negativism, when the patient has been led to the toilet but relaxes the sphincters so soon as he leaves it. A constant feature is a *thinking disorder*. On recovery memory is largely a blank even for striking experiences during the psychosis and, when accessible during the stupor to any questioning, a failure of intellectual functions is apparent. An *ideational content* may be gathered while the stupor is incubating, during interruptions, or from the recollections of recovered patients. Its peculiarity is a preoccupation with the theme of death, which is not merely a dominant topic but, often, an exclusive interest. Probably to be related to this is a tendency, present in some cases, to sudden suicidal impulses, that are as apparently planless and unexpected as the conduct of many catatonics. Finally the disease is prone to exhibit certain *physical* peculiarities. A low fever [236] is common and so are skin and circulatory anomalies. A loss of weight is the rule, and menstruation is almost always suppressed.

As to the frequency of stupor no figures are available, for the simple reason that the diagnosis in large clinics has not been made with sufficient accuracy to justify any statistics. Most of these cases are usually called catatonia, depression, allied to manic-depressive insanity or allied to dementia præcox. The majority of the stupors reported in this book were in women, but this is merely the result of chance, since it has been easier in the Psychiatric Institute to study functional psychoses in the female division, while the male ward has been reserved largely for organic psychoses. The majority of the patients seem to be between 15 and 25 years of age, so that it is, presumably, a reaction of youthful years. In our experience most cases occur among the lower classes, which agrees with the opinion of Wilmanns who found this tendency among prisoners.

This gives a brief description of the deep stupor. But even our typical cases did not present this picture during the entire psychosis. They showed phases when, superficially viewed, they were not in stupor but suffered from the above symptoms as tendencies rather than states. There are also many psychoses where complete stupor is never developed. This gives us our justification for speaking of the *stupor reaction*, which consists of these symptoms (or most of them) no matter in how slight a [237] degree they may be present. The analogy to mania and hypomania is compelling. The latter is merely a dilution of the former. Both are forms of the manic reaction. We consequently regard stupor and partial stupor as different degrees of the same psychotic process which we term the stupor reaction. To understand it the symptoms should be separately analyzed and then correlated.

The most fundamental characteristic of the stupor symptoms is the change in affect which can be summed up in one word — apathy.

It is fundamental because it seems as if the symptoms built around apathy constitute the stupor reaction. The emotional poverty is evidenced by a lack of feeling, loss of energy and an absence of the normal urge of living. This is quite different from the emotional blocking of the retarded depression, for in the latter the patient shows either by speech or facial expression a definite suffering. The tendency to reduction of affect produces two effects on such emotions as internal ideas or environmental events may stimulate. Exhibitions of emotion are either reduced or dissociated. For instance, anxiety is frequently diminished to an expression of dazed bewilderment; or, isolated and partial exhibitions of mood occur, as when laughter, tears or blushing are seen as quite isolated symptoms. This latter—the dissociation of affect—seems to occur only in stupor and dementia præcox. It should be noted, however, that inappropriateness of affect is never observed in a true benign stupor. A final peculiarity is the tendency to [238] interruption of the apathetic habit, when the patient may return to life, as it were, for a few moments and then relapse.

Closely related to the apathy, and probably merely an expression of it, is the inactivity which is both muscular and mental. It exists in all gradations from that of flaccidity of voluntary muscles, with relaxation of the sphincters, and from states where there is complete absence of any evidence of mentation to conditions of mere physical and psychic slowness. After recovery the stupor patient frequently speaks of having felt dead, paralyzed or drugged.

By far the commonest cause of emotional expression or interruption in the inactivity is negativism. This is a perversity of behavior which seems to express antagonism to the environment or to the wishes of those about the patient. In the partial stupors it is seen as active opposition and cantankerousness. In the more profound conditions it is represented by muscular resistiveness or rigidity, or refusal to swallow food when placed in the mouth. Occasionally, too, the patient may even in a deep stupor retain urine so long that catheterization is necessary. All the explanations which one may gather from the patients' own utterances, mainly retrospective, seem to point to negativism expressing a desire to be left alone. The appearance of perverse behavior in aimless striking or mere muscular rigidity seems to be an example of dissociation of affect.

[239]

Catalepsy is an important symptom because, although it occurred in slightly less than a third of our cases, it seems to be a peculiarity of the stupor reaction found but rarely in other benign psychoses. It seems never to occur without there being some evidence of mental activity, and, consequently, we are forced to conclude that it is of mental rather than of physical origin. Just what it means psychically it is impossible to state without much more extended observations. We conjecture tentatively, however, that the retention of fixed positions is in part merely a phenomenon of perseveration, and in part an acceptance of what the patient takes to be a command from the examiner, and sometimes a distorted form of muscular resistiveness.

The intellectual processes suffer more seriously in stupor than in any other form of manic-depressive insanity. Not only do the deep stupors betray no evidence of mentation during the acme of the psychosis, but retrospectively they usually speak of their minds being a blank. Incompleteness and slowness of intellectual operations are highly characteristic features of the partial stupors and of the incubation period of the more profound reactions. The features of this defect are a difficulty in grasping the nature of the environment, a slowness in elaborating what impressions are received, with resulting disorientation, poor performance of any set tests and incomplete memory for external events when recovery has taken place. At times the thinking disorder may develop with great suddenness or [240] improve as quickly, and a tendency to isolated evidences of mental acuity is another example of the inconsistency which is so highly characteristic of stupor. We should note, however, that these sporadic exhibitions of mentality are always associated with brief emotional awakening.

When we turn to examine the fragmentary utterances of stupor patients, we are surprised by the narrowness and uniformity of the ideational content. It seems to be confined to thoughts of death or closely related conceptions. Thirty-five out of thirty-six consecutive cases at one time or another referred literally to death. It is commonest during the onset, as all but five of these patients spoke of it during the incubation of their psychoses. Hence we conclude that death ideas and stupor are consecutive phenomena in the same fundamental process. As two-thirds of the series interrupted the stupor to speak of death or to attempt suicide, we assume that this relationship persists. Only a quarter gave any retrospective account of these fancies, so we presume that their psychotic experiences were repressed with recovery.

The usual form in which the idea appears is as a delusion of going to die or, literally, of being dead. It may appear as being in Heaven or Hell. A theoretically important group is that which includes the patients who, in addition, speak of being in situations such as under the water or underground, which we have mythological and psychological evidence to believe are formulations of a rebirth [241] fantasy. Not rarely, preoccupation with death is expressed in sudden impulsive suicidal attempts.

The affective setting of these different formulations is important. A delusion of literal death occurs with complete apathy. The wish to die is apt to appear without the usual accompaniment of sadness or distress but still with considerable energy when impulsive suicidal attempts are made. A prospect of death, particularly when there is anticipation of being killed, is apt in manic-depressive insanity to occur in a setting of anxiety. Similarly one ordinarily observes fear in the patient who has delusions of drowning or burial. In the stupor cases, however, this painful affect seems to be reduced to a mere dazed bewilderment or feeble exhibitions of a desire for safety, such as the slow swimming movements of a patient who thought she was under the water. When these ideas of danger become allied to everyday interests—husband or child imperiled, etc.—a weak affect in the form of depression is apt to occur.

Physical symptoms are more common than in any other benign psychosis. Of these the most nearly constant is a low fever, the temperature running between 99° and 101°. Twenty-eight out of thirty-five cases had this slight elevation with a tendency for it to occur immediately at the beginning of marked stupor symptoms. Although the evidence does not positively exclude any possibility of infection, it speaks distinctly against this view. A possible explanation is that the low fever is a secondary symp [242] tom. The suprarenal glands may function insufficiently as a consequence of the emotional poverty, since all emotions which have been experimentally studied seem to stimulate the production of adrenalin. Without this normal hormone for the activity of the sympathetic nervous system, there would be a disturbance of skin and circulatory reactions that would interfere with the normal heat loss. Suggestive evidence to support this view comes from the frequency with which the extremities are cyanotic or cold, the skin greasy, sweating profuse or absent, and so on. Further observations are necessary to confirm or disprove this hypothesis, but we feel inclined to accept it tentatively because it is plausible and consistent with the view that stupor is essentially a psychogenic type of reaction. Another physical anomaly, which is presumably of endocrine origin, is the suppression of the menses. This probably results from lowered nutrition. In some cases it ensues directly on a psychic crisis before any nutritional change can have taken place. Finally, among the symptoms of possible physical origin, epileptoid attacks were described in two of our cases. This is chiefly of interest in that such phenomena are extremely rare in the benign psychoses.

We believe that the mental symptoms summarized above constitute a specific psychotic type of reaction capable of appearing in any severity from mere lethargy and indifference to profound stupor. Since the prognosis is good, we feel obliged to classify this with the manic-depressive reactions. Further justi [243] fication for this grouping is found in the occurrence of the stupor reaction as a phase in many manic-depressive psychoses. A patient may swing from mania to stupor as from mania to depression, and when the partial stupors are recognized as milder forms of the same process, it seems to be a frequent type of reaction.

If stupor be a reaction type, its laws must be psychological. According to the view of modern psychopathology, the essence of insanity is regression with indolent thinking as opposed to progressive and energetic mentation. One can look on stupor as being a profound regression. Effort is abandoned (apathy and inactivity), while the ideational content expresses a desire for a retreat from the world in death. It is possible to think of this regression as a return to the mental habit of the suckling period, when spontaneous effort is at its minimum. This, too, is the time when petulance and tantrums are frequent expression of a wish to be left alone, which may account for the negativism as a consistent symptom of the same regressive progress.

Just as we regress in sleep, to rise refreshed for a new day's duties, so the stupor case often shows excessive energy in a hypomanic phase before complete normality is reached. This corresponds again to the age-old association of the ideas of death and rebirth which we see together so frequently in stupor. It is the psychology of wiping the slate clean for a fresh start.

The development and symptoms of stupor furnish [244] evidence in support of the hypothesis of this type of regression. Dissatisfaction of any kind is the setting in which the psychosis begins and the commonest precipitating factor is some reminder of death. That loss of energy appears with the stupor is evident from the inactivity and apathy, while the thinking disorder can be shown to be the result of the same loss. The different "levels" of the stupor reaction also conform to a theory of regression. First there is mere indifference and quietness; then appear false ideas when normality is so far abandoned as to mean a loss of the sense of reality; withdrawal of interest from the environment, with its consequent centering of self, leads to the next stage—that of the spoiled child reaction; then follows the exclusion of the world around in the dramatization of death; finally, in the deepest stupor, mentation is so far abandoned that we can gather no evidence of even this delusion being present.

Atypical features in stupor have to do mainly with interruptions, interludes as it were, of elation, anxiety or perplexity. These are explicable as awakenings from the nothingness of stupor into imaginations such as characterize the other manic-depressive psychoses. When such tendencies are present, the co-existence of the stupor process may tone down the emotional response or prevent its complete repression so that insufficient or dissociated affects appear. A combination of the stupor tendency to apathy with the mood of another reac [245] tion is probably the only combination of affects to be met with in psychiatry.

The stupor reaction, then, is a simple regression, with a limitation of energy, emotion and ideational content, the last being confined to notions of death. All functional psychoses are regressions. How do the others differ from this? We need only answer this question in so far as it concerns the clinical states resembling benign stupors. Stupors occur frequently in catatonic dementia præcox. In this disease there is a regression of interest to primitive fantastic thoughts, and with this a perversion of energy and emotion. This corrupts the purity of the stupor picture so that inconsistencies, such as empty giggling, atypical delusions and scattered speech, occur. Other impurities are to be found in the frequent orientation of the dementia præcox stupor patient which is discovered to be astonishingly good, or in free speech associated with apathy and inactivity. Such symptoms usually appear quite early and should enable one to make a positive diagnosis within a short time after patient comes under observation. As a matter of fact, in many if not most cases there is a slow onset characterized by the pathognomonic symptoms of dementia præcox before the actual stupor sets in.

Other psychoses superficially resembling stupor are the perplexity and absorbed manic (manic stupor) states. We have reason to believe that both these conditions are essentially the result of absorption in kaleidoscopic ideas. Their appearance [246] is that of inactivity and indifference to the outside world, just as a dreamer seems placid and apathetic. But these reactions are not without emotion which may sometimes be obvious, and the richness of the mental content is sooner or later manifest.

Finally, from a practical standpoint, an important peculiarity of benign stupor is the tendency for response to stimulation in amelioration of the process. Close attention to these patients is advisable, therefore, not merely for the sake of their physical health, but also because any attention tends to keep them mentally alive or revive their waning energy. Visits of relations often initiate recovery in a striking way. From occurrences such as these, psychiatrists should gain hints for valuable therapeutic experiments.

So much for the technical, psychiatric aspects of the stupor problem. We have frequently spoken of it, however, as a psychobiological reaction. If this be a sound view, similar tendencies should appear in everyday life, the psychotic phenomena being merely the exaggerations of a fundamental type of human and animal behavior. Shamming of death in the face of danger and animal catalepsy come to mind at once, but since we know nothing of the associated affective states we should be chary of using them even as analogies. We are on safer ground in discussing problems of human psychology.

It is evident that there are psychological parallels between the stupor reaction and sleep, while future work may show physiological similarities as well. [247] Apathy towards the environment, inactivity and a thinking disorder are common to both. But sleep reactions do not occur in bed alone. Weariness produces indifference, physical sluggishness, inattention and a mild thinking disorder such as are seen in partial stupors. The phenomena of the midday nap are strikingly like those of stupor. The individual who enjoys this faculty has a facility for retiring from the world psychologically and as a result of this psychic release is capable of renewed activity (analogous to post-stuporous hypomania) that cannot be the result of physiological repair, since the whole affair may last for only a few minutes.

In everyday life there are more protracted states where the comparison can also be made. When life fails to yield us what we want, we tend to become bored—a condition of apathy and inactivity, forming a nice parallel to stupor inasmuch as external reminders of reality and demands for activity are apt to call out irritability. A form of what is really mental disease, although not called insanity, is permanent boredom, a deterioration of interest, energy and even intelligence by which many troubled souls solve their problems. A sudden withdrawal from the world we call stupor. When the same thing happens insidiously, the condition is labeled according to the financial and social status of the victim. He is a bum, a loafer, a mendicant or, more politely, a disillusioned recluse. Frequently this undiagnosed dement has satisfied himself with a weak, cynical philosophy that life is not worth while.

[248]

It is but a step from valueless life to death and the same tendency which makes the patient fancy he is dead, leads the tired man to sleep, the poet to sigh in verse for dissolution, and the myth maker to fabricate rebirth. The religions of the world are full of this yearning, which reaches its purest expression in the belief and philosophy of Nirvana. The ideational content of stupor has also its analogue in crime. The desire for perpetuation of relationships unprosperous in this world is not seen only in the delusion of mutual death. One can hardly pick up a newspaper without reading of some unhappy man or woman who has slain a disillusioned lover and then committed suicide.

Footnotes:

[12] Kirby, George H.: "The Catatonic Syndrome and Its Relation to Manic-Depressive Insanity." *Jour. of Nervous and Mental Disease*, Vol. XL, No. 11, 1913.

CHAPTER XV
THE LITERATURE OF STUPOR [C]

The cases of benign stupor which we report here are not clinical curiosities. Taking the symptoms as the products of a reaction type, the latter is really quite common. One, therefore, asks what other psychiatrists have done with this material. How have they described these stupors, how classified them? This chapter, essentially an appendix, attempts to give a brief answer to this inquiry. No attempt is made to catalogue all that has been written on or around this subject but only to mention typical reports and viewpoints.

The French, beginning with Pinel in the 18th Century, were the first to write extensively of stupor. An excellent paper by Dagonet [13] appeared in 1872, in which such literature as had appeared up to that time is discussed. He defines "Stupidity" as a form of insanity in which "delirious" ideas may or may not be present, which has for its characteristic symptoms a state of more or less manifest [250] stupor and a greater or less incapacity to coördinate ideas, to elaborate sensations experienced and accomplish voluntary acts necessary for adaptation. This would seem to include our "partial stupor," as well as the more marked cases.

He quotes an excellent definition from Louyer Villermay (Dict. des sc. méd. t. LIII, p. 67). "Stupor is a term applied to stupefaction of the brain. It is recognizable by the diminution or enfeeblement of internal sensation and by a greater difficulty in exercising memory, judgment and imagination. It is accompanied by a general numbness and a weakness of feeling and movement. The patient, then, has an indefinite and stupid expression, he understands questions put to him with difficulty, and answers them with effort or not at all. He seems overwhelmed with sleep, he forgets to withdraw his tongue after showing it to the doctor, he complains of no uncomfortable sensation, of no illness, he seems to take no interest in what goes on about him.... The stupor patient is a fool who does not speak, in this being more tolerable than the one who speaks [delightful naiveté!]. One who is dumbfounded by surprise or fright is also to be called stuporous."

Dagonet says stupor results from various causes, such as exhaustion, or emotional and intellectual factors. Clinically it varies in kind and degree according to the situation in which it develops. When it develops during normal mental health, it disappears when its cause does. In insanity it appears in the course of a psychosis of some duration, of [251] which it seems a part, an exaggeration of some symptom of the general condition. Evidently he views stupor as a type of reaction: as a more or less complete suspension of the operation of intellectual faculties, a more or less sudden subtraction of nervous forces. This reaction can result from a fright or the memory of it, a brain lesion or trauma, the action of narcotics, exhausting fevers, excessive grief, the terrors of alcoholic hallucinations, epileptic seizures, profound anemia and nervous exhaustion consequent on sexual excess. He is careful to say that both symptoms and treatment vary with the varied etiologies.

He credits Pinel with being the first to call attention to stupor. This author claimed that some persons with extreme sensibility could be so upset by any violent emotion as to have their faculties suspended or obliterated. He noted, too, that stupors frequently terminated in manic phases of 20 to 30 days' duration. Pinel also emphasized the apathy of these cases. Esquirol called stupor "acute dementia," a term which persisted in French literature for a long time. He described an interesting circular case where alternations between mania and typical stupor took place. He mentions too the dangerous, impulsive tendencies of many patients. Georget emphasized the fact which Pinel had also noted, that retrospectively the stupor patient says his mind was a blank during the attack. In 1835 Etoc-Demazy published on the subject. He regarded stupor not as a separate form of insanity [252] but a complication ensuing on monomania or mania. He recognized the partial as well as complete stupor. He thought the condition was due to cerebral edema, as did other writers of that period. Dagonet remarks about this last—a lesson not learned in fifty years by the profession—that demonstrable edema does *not* produce the typical symptoms of stupor. Baillarger in 1843 (Annales Médico-psychologiques) was the first whose ambition to simplify psychiatric types led to denial of a separate kind of reaction. He claimed that stupor was not a form of insanity but an extension of a "délire mélancholique." As Dagonet remarks, every symptom by which he characterizes stupor is a psychiatric symptom and insanity can consist just as well in the diminution as the perversion or exaltation of normal faculties. Some of Baillarger's cases had false ideas, some apparently none at all. Dagonet thinks this justifies two types, one a dream-like state and another where no ideas are present, although he admits one may be an exaggeration of the other. Brierre de Boismont (Annales Médico-psychologique, 1851, p. 442) compares these two kinds of stupors to deep sleep when intelligence is completely suspended and to sleep with dreams. (These two types would correspond to our "absorbed mania" and true deep stupor.) He urges strongly the separation of stupor from melancholia as an entirely different type of reaction, in this connection citing the views pro and con of various authors. Of these [253] Delasiauve is particularly cogent in discriminating stupor from melancholia on the grounds of the difference of the emotional reactions and of the intellectual disorder and the real paucity of thought in the former psychosis.

After quoting these and other authors, Dagonet offers an explanation for the diversity of opinion. He says that stupor following another psychosis may retain some of its symptoms, so that a mixture obtains, as often in medicine. He then gives excellent descriptions of three types: the deep stupor with paralysis of the faculties, the cases that are absorbed in false ideas, and ecstatic cataleptics.

The remainder of his paper is concerned with cases and discussions about them. He cites examples of stupor following fear or other emotional shocks, following grave injuries such as the loss of a limb, following head trauma and with typhoid fever. As to the last he points out that delirious features are prominent. Many authors have assigned sexual excesses as a cause of stupor. The psychosis, Dagonet says, is not pure but more a mixture of hypochondria and depression. Relationship with mania is next considered. He says that stupor may succeed, alternate with or precede mania. His cases seem mainly to have been what we call absorbed manics or manic stupors. In fact, he uses the last term. The commonest introductory psychosis, he claims, is depression, but from his brief case reports it would seem that most of his [254] patients were not stuporous, in the narrow sense of the term, but severely retarded depressions. In fact, in perusing his case material comprising "stupors" in the course of many types of functional insanity, or as a complication of epilepsy or general paralysis, it is evident that in practice he does not follow the discriminative definitions of the earlier portion of his paper. For him, apparently, patients who are markedly inaccessible to examination from whatever cause are "stuporous." He closes with excellent remarks on physical and psychic treatment. As to prognosis he has nothing to say beyond the opinion that most of the cases recover.

If Dagonet be accepted as summarizing the early French work, we can conclude that their generalizations were on the whole quite sound. These were: that stupor is an abnormal mental reaction, usually psychogenic but often the result of exhaustion, that it consists in a paralysis of emotion, will and intelligence; that the prognosis is usually good; that mental stimulation may produce recovery. What remained to be done after this work was the refinement in detail of these generalizations, particularly in respect to the differentiation of prognostically benign and malignant types. But other Frenchmen did not take up this work, apparently, for the brilliant psychopathologists of the next generations attended to stupor only in so far as it was hysterical.

An Englishman, however, soon took up the task, adding more exactness to his formulations. New [255] ington [14] published his important paper in 1874. A nascent stage of stupor, he thinks, is a common reaction to great exhaustion, "such as hard mental work, prolonged or acute illness, dissipation, etc." Such conditions, like the grave psychotic forms, he regarded as due to physical exhaustion of the brain cells, but, since he thought psychic stress could produce this exhaustion, this "organic" view did not bias his general formulations. He makes a division into two stupors: Anergic Stupor and Delusional Stupor. The former may be primary, being generally caused by a sudden intense shock (Esquirol's "Acute Dementia"), or secondary (a) to convulsions of any kind, (b) to mania in women, (c) to any other prolonged nervous exhaustion. The delusional form results from (a) intense melancholia, (b) from general paralysis in which it may be intercurrent, (c) from epileptic seizures. When one examines his points of difference between these two types, it becomes clear that Newington really gave an excellent differentiation of benign and malignant stupor—in fact, it is the only serious attempt at such discrimination prior to this present work. What is more remarkable is the fact that, although he clearly saw the clinical differences, he failed to see that the two types differed prognostically. His description is given in a table sufficiently concise to justify its quotation *in extenso*.

[256]

	ANERGIC STUPOR	DELUSIONAL STUPOR
Etiology —	Hereditary and individual liability to sudden loss of *vis nervosa*.	Hereditary.
Onset —	Rapid.	Usually insidious, may be almost instantaneous.
Symptoms —	Intellect greatly impaired.	Conduct shows reasoning power.
Memory —	Seems to be swept away as far as possible.	Found after recovery to have been preserved to a great extent.
Emotional Capacity —	Nil or almost so. Tears frequent but due to relaxation of sphincter muscles. Features relaxed, eyes vacant and not constantly fixed.	Evidence of grief, fear, etc., in facial expressions and wringing and clasping of hands. Tears rare. Great contraction of features [grimacing?]. Eyes fixed on one point, usually upwards or downwards, or else obstinately closed.
Volition —	Almost absent.	Frequently great stubbornness, refusal to do what is wanted. On the other hand, intense determination in following out own plan.
Motor System —	Weak and uncertain. Patient has to be led about and if placed on a	But little interfered with, independently of sheer asthenia, produced by

	seat or in some position does not move. ("Cataleptoid" condition.)	patient's conduct. May stand behind door or kneel on floor in constrained position even for days.
[257] *Sensory System* *Reflex System —*	} Both dull.	Ditto. There seems to be a much greater ability to bear severe pain.
Pupils —	Dilated.	Tendency to contraction.
Sleep —	Generally good.	Intense sleeplessness.
General bodily condition —	Emaciation, sometimes extreme, usually rapid, with rapid recovery of flesh. Often not much loss of weight, though whole tone is lowered.	Affected *pari passu* with mental state and seems governed by it.
Vascular System —	Pulse slow, sometimes almost imperceptible. Cyanotic appearance, edema and iciness of extremities. Great decrease of vitality in peripheral structures, as shown by asthenic eruptions and production of vermin.	Pulse weak and often quick and thready. Complexion anemic and sallow. The other appearances may be present but come on later and are less marked.
Digestive System —	Tongue clean or if furred it is moist. Appetite *apathetic*, bowels not irregular, but habits very dirty.	Tongue dry, small and furred. Refusal of food. Great constipation. Dirtiness of habits rare.

If one compares these data with those given in the chapter on Malignant Stupors, it is seen that in the main Newington has made the same discrimination as we have. He is certainly wrong in denying "negativism" to his anergic type. Probably, too, he attempts too fine a distinction between the [258] physical symptoms of the two groups. His conclusions are interesting: that in the anergic cases there is an *absence* of cerebration, while amongst the delusional there is an abnormal *presence* of intense but perverted cerebration. This is not unlike our own view. He thinks the difference in memory is the most important differential point. Sex is important in determining the nature of the stupor, for he found the anergic type following mania in females only. He observed such an end to manic attacks in 6 out of 36 cases. All his cases were under 30 and he regards the prognosis as good on the whole. As to treatment he emphasizes the necessity for "moral pressure" as a stimulus and cites a case of rapid improvement after a change of scene.

Since 1874 very little advance has been made by British psychiatrists, as seen by a perusal of Clouston's [15] summary in 1904. He regards sex exhaustion as a highly frequent cause, although Dagonet had shown 32 years before that sex abuse does not produce a true stupor. He thinks stupor usually follows depression or mania and says that "the 'Confusional Insanity' of German and American authors is just a lesser degree of stupor." Omitting his stupors in general paralysis and epilepsy he makes three clinical divisions: *melancholic or conscious stupor*, which is not a product of delusions, although delusions of death or great wickedness may be present, impulsiveness and fits may be observed; *anergic or [259] unconscious stupor*, which corresponds roughly to our deep, benign stupor; and *secondary stupor* after acute mental disease, which resembles our partial stupor. He warns against a rash diagnosis of dementia in this last group. His views on the importance of mental causation and the relation to manic-depressive insanity may be gathered from these sentences: "The condition of the mental portion of the convolutions in stupor is probably analogous to the stupidity of a nervous child when terrified or bullied." "Stupor is frequently one of the stages of alternating insanity following the exalted condition. It is more apt to occur in those where the exalted period is acutely maniacal. The stupor is usually melancholic in form." Since he claims that the anergic is a "very curable form of mental disease," while only 50% of the melancholic cases recover, it seems clear that this division is not prognostically final. The "melancholic" is evidently Newington's "delusional" without his more accurate discrimination of symptoms.

From the standpoint of accurate description the opinion may be ventured that there is a gap in the literature from the early French writers and Newington up to the paper by Kirby, which has been discussed in the first chapter. This gap is filled by literature of the German schools and their adherents in other countries. German psychiatry has been concerned mainly with classification or the elaborate examination of certain symptoms. Inevitably such a program militates against detached objective clini [260] cal description. It is hard to record symptoms that interfere with classification. German psychiatry has tended to make the insane patient a type rather than an individual. Hence the gap in the descriptive literature of stupor.

The necessity of establishing the possibility of some stupors having a good prognosis has arisen from Kraepelin's work. He can rightly be viewed as the father of modern psychiatry because he introduced a classification based on syndromes and taught us to recognize these disease groups in their early stages. Inevitably with such an ambitious scheme as the pigeon-holing of all psychotic phenomena some mistakes were made. Most of these appear in the border zone between dementia præcox and manic-depressive insanity. The latter group being narrowly defined, the former had to be a waste basket containing whatever did not seem to be a purely emotional reaction. Clinical experience soon proved that many cases which, according to Kraepelin's formulæ, were in the dementia præcox group, recovered. Adolf Meyer was one of the first to protest and offered categories of "Allied to Manic-Depressive Insanity" or "Allied to Dementia Præcox," as tentative diagnostic classifications to include the doubtful cases.

Difficulties with stupor furnish an excellent example of the confusion which results from the adoption of rigid terminology. The earlier psychiatrists were free to regard a patient in stupor as capable of recovery as well as deterioration. When Kahl [261] baum included stupor with "Catatonia," the situation was not changed, for he did not claim a hopeless prognosis for this group. But when Kraepelin made catatonia a subdivision of dementia præcox, all stupors (except obvious phases of manic-depressive insanity) had to be hysterical or malignant. Faced with this dilemma psychiatrists have either called recoveries "remissions" or, like E. Meyer, claimed that one-fifth or one-fourth of catatonics really get well.

As a matter of fact it seems clear that stupor is a psychobiological reaction that can occur in settings of quite varied clinical conditions. It is not necessary to detail publications describing stupors in hysteria, epilepsy, dementia præcox or in the organic psychoses. It may be of interest, however, to cite some examples of acute, benign stupors and the discussion of them which appear in the literature of recent years.

An important group is that of stupors occurring as prison psychoses. Stern [16] mentions that acute stupors are found in this group. Wilmanns [17] examined the records for five years in a prison and discovered that there were two forms of psychotic reaction, a paranoid and a stupor type. It is interesting psychologically that the former appeared largely among prisoners in solitary confinement, while the stupors developed preponderantly among those who were not isolated. The stupors recovered more quickly. He describes the psychosis thus: The prisoner becomes rather suddenly excited, destructive and assaultive; then soon passes into an inactive state, where he lies in bed, mute, with open expressionless eyes. He is clean, however; eats spontaneously and attends to his own hygienic needs. Some cases are roused by transport from the jail to the hospital but sink into lethargy again when they reach their beds. Physically, they show disturbances of sensation which vary from analgesia to hypesthesia. There are a rapid pulse, positive Romberg sign, exaggerated reflexes, fibrillary twitching of the tongue and tremor of the hands. Recovery takes place gradually. They begin to react to physical stimuli and to answer questions, although still inhibited, until consciousness is quite clear. When speech begins, it is found that they are usually disoriented for place and time as the result of an amnesia which sets in sharply with the excitement. This memory defect gradually improves *pari passu* with the other symptoms.

Two attacks in the same prisoner of what seem to have been typical stupor are reported by Kutner [18] and Chotzen. [19] The patient was a recidivist of unstable mental make-up. At the age of 34 he was sent to prison for three years. Shortly after confinement began, he became stuporous, being mute and negativistic, soiling, refusing food and showing stereotypy. On being shifted to another institution he appeared suddenly much better, although he remained apathetic and dull for some months. A striking feature was a complete amnesia, not merely for the stupor but also for his trial and entrance to the prison. At the age of 42, he was again incarcerated. A practically identical picture again developed, with recovery when his environment was changed, and with a similar amnesia. Recovery seemed to be complete and there were no hysterical stigmata. The interesting features of this case are that a typical stupor seems to have been precipitated by imprisonment, while the retroactive amnesia covering a painful period of the patient's life reminds one of hysteria.

A case which is more difficult to interpret is reported briefly by Seelig. [20] A man of 20 with bad inheritance tried to steal 100 marks. When sent to jail he became ill shortly before his trial was due and was sent to a hospital. There he seemed anxious, was shy, and gave slow answers, with initial lip motions and had to be urged to take hold of objects. All this sounds more like a pure depression than a stupor. But he also had paralogia. This might make one think of a Ganser reaction on the background of depression. S., however, calls it an [264] hysterical stupor, although he agreed with Moeli that it was hard to differentiate from a catatonic state.

Löwenstein [21] reports an interesting case of a dégénéré who had had hysterical attacks. He suddenly developed stupor symptoms, which lasted with interruptions for nearly two years. After recovery and during the interruptions the patient explained his mutism, refusal to swallow, his filthiness and general negativism as all occasioned by delusions. He was commanded by God to act thus, the attendants were devils, and so on. He spoke, too, of being under hypnotic influence. In addition there were other delusions such as that he had killed his brother. The attack came on with the belief that he was going to die, otherwise none of the ideas were typical of the stupors we have studied. Another incongruous symptom was that he did not seem to be really apathetic, he reacted constantly to the environment. The author comments on the absence of senseless motor phenomena, such as would be expected in a "catatonic." His complete memory of the psychosis also speaks against the usual form of stupor. It seems possible that this psychosis was neither hysterical nor a benign stupor in our sense, but, rather, an acute schizophrenic reaction such as one occasionally sees. From the account which Löwenstein gives, one gathers that the patient was absorbed in a wealth of imaginations.

[265]

Gregor [22] tells of a stupor which is unusual in that it consisted only of symptoms connected with inactivity, which did not affect the intellectual processes. The patient was a rubber worker who suddenly developed a depression with self-accusation and convulsions. She was soon admitted to a clinic and then showed mutism and catalepsy. Later she became totally immobile with no apparent psychic reactions, and soiled. Gregor studied pulse, respiration and respiratory volume in their reflex manifestations and found nothing unusual. Next he tried to discover if there were voluntary alterations in respiration. He discovered that the respiratory curve could be changed by calling out words to her, by odors associated with suggestions, menaces, etc. [This is suggestive of the dissociation of affect, which we have discussed.] After two months she recovered, *with complete recollection of the stupor period.* It was then proven that the absence of reactions was not the same as the lack of perception of stimuli.

Froederström [23] reports a case that suggests hysteria, where the stupor lasted for 32 years. A girl at the age of 14 fell on the ice, had a headache, went to bed and stayed there for 32 years. She lay there [266] immobile, occasionally spoke briefly and took nourishment, when it was put at a definite place at the edge of the bed. At first (according to a late statement of her brothers) this consisted only of water but was soon changed to two glasses of milk a day. After being in this state for ten years she was placed in a hospital for two weeks, where she was mute, did not react to pin pricks and had to be fed. It seems that at home she secretly looked after herself, for she kept her hair and nails in condition. Sometimes she sat up and stared at the ceiling.

After attending to the patient for 30 years, her mother died. The patient cried for several days when told of it, and after this she took nourishment of her own accord. Two years later a brother died.

Again she cried on hearing the news. Her father, who looked after her when the mother was dead, also died. Then a governess came into the home, who noticed that furniture was moved about when she was alone.

At the age of 46 she suddenly woke up and asked at once for her mother. She claimed total amnesia for the period of her stupor, including the stay at the hospital. She could summon memories of her childhood, however. Her brothers she did not recognize and said, "They must be small." She recalled the fall on the ice and coming home with headache, toothache and pain in the back. Her general knowledge was limited but she could read and write. Her expression and appearance was that of a young person, only her atrophic breasts and the [267] fat on her buttocks betraying her age. She had been well for four years at the time the report was made.

He thinks that a certain tendency to exaggeration and simulation speak for hysteria. We would be more inclined to view the fact that she looked after herself in spite of complete amnesia as evidence of hysteria.

Another protracted case suggestive of hysteria is that reported by Gadelius. [24] The patient was a tailor, 32 years old, who had always been rather taciturn and slow. A year before admission he began to have ideas of persecution and to shun people. Then he developed a stereotyped response, "It is nice weather," whenever he was addressed. A month before admission inactivity set in. He would sit immobile in his chair with closed eyes and relaxed face; he resisted when an attempt was made to put him to bed. His color was pale.

He was taken to hospital on November 1, 1882, where he was observed to be immobile and to have little reaction to pin pricks. When a limb was raised, it fell limply. However, he would leave bed to go to the toilet. Tube-feeding became necessary, but when the tube was inserted in his nose, he woke up. He then showed an amnesia not merely for his illness but for his whole life: he did not know his father, that he was married or that he had a mother. To [268] wards the end of November, he became limp again and answered, "I don't know" to most questions. In December, however, he improved again and for a few months these variations occurred.

From April, 1883, to May, 1886, he was in deep stupor, almost absolutely immobile and close to being completely anesthetic even with strong Faradic currents. Towards the end of this period he walked about *whenever he thought he was not watched.* He was very cautious about this and became motionless any time he became aware of observation. (Gadelius thinks this was not simulation but the expression of an automatism on the basis of a vague fixed idea.)

This condition persisted apparently for five years more, by the end of which time the anesthesia had turned into a hyperesthesia. A year later he began to eat. It was now found that he had an amnesia for his illness and former life, so that he did not even recognize a needle or pair of scissors. He knew that he was born in the month of February and retained some facility in calculation, in speech, walking and usual motions. Then he regained all his memories and resumed his trade as tailor. He was discharged in June, 1893, nearly eleven years after admission.

It seems safe to say that elements at least of hysteria appear in this history, such as the profound retroactive amnesia and appearance of simulation in the conduct of the patient. Accurate and rapid grasp of the environment is necessary for such a watch as he kept on the eye of his attendants. Men [269] tal acuity of this grade combined with amnesia looks more like an hysterical than a manic-depressive process.

Leroy [25] describes a case much like ours which is interesting from a therapeutic standpoint. The patient was a woman who passed from a severe depression with hallucinations and anxiety into a long stupor, from which she recovered completely. There was no negativism and no affect, although the latter appeared so soon as contact began to be established. When well she had a complete amnesia for the onset of the psychosis. Leroy attributed the recovery, in part at least, to the thorough attention given the patient. Kraepelinian rigidity is seen, however, in the author's refusal to regard the case as "circular" because of the lack of all cyclic symptoms. He takes refuge in the meaningless label "Mental Confusion."

An important group of cases is that of the stupors occurring during warfare. Considering stupor as a withdrawal reaction, it is surprising there were so few of them, although partial stupor reactions as functional perpetuation of concussion were very common. The editor saw several typical cases in young children in London who passed into long "sleeps" apparently as a result of the air raids. [270] Myers [26] has given us the best account of stupors in actual warfare. A typical case was that of a man who was found in a dazed condition and difficult to arouse. He could give little information about himself, could neither read nor write and never spoke voluntarily. A week later his speech was still limited and labored and no account of recent events could be obtained from him. Under hypnosis he was induced to talk of the accident which had precipitated this disorder. He became excited in telling his story, evidently visualizing many of the events. In several successive séances, more data were obtained and a cure effected. Myers points out that in all his cases there was a mental condition which varied from slight depression to actual stupor, all had amnesias of variable extent and all had headaches. The mental content seemed to be confined to thoughts of bombardment, with a tendency for the mind always to wander to this topic. The author thinks that pain is a guardian protecting the patient from too distressing thoughts. An effort to speak would cause pain in the throat of a case of mutism and, sometimes, when a distressing memory was sought after under hypnosis, physical pain would wake the sleeper. His view is that pains tend to preserve the mutism and amnesia, so that there are "inhibitory processes" causing the stupor, which prevent the patient from further suffering. He does [271] not find either in theory or experience reason to believe that these conditions are the result of either suggestion or "fixed ideas." He thinks it natural that the last symptom of the stupor to disappear should be mutism, as speech and vision are the prime factors in communicating with environment. [As has been noted frequently in this book, mutism is a common residual symptom of the benign stupor.] Myers believes that in nearly every instance mutism follows stupor and is merely an attenuation of the latter process. When deafness is associated with mutism, he thinks it is often due merely to the inattention of the stuporous state.

In this connection we should mention that Gucci [27] points out that stupor patients with mutism of long duration may, when requested, read fluently and then relapse again into complete unreactiveness towards auditory impressions. This, we would say, is probably an example of a more or less automatic intellectual operation occurring when the patient is sufficiently stimulated, although he cannot be raised to the point of spontaneous verbal productivity.

As these scattered reports about benign stupors are so unsatisfactory, one naturally turns to text-books. Little more appears in them. Kraepelin treats stupors occurring in manic-depressive insanity as falling into two groups, the depressive and [272] manic. The former seems to be nearer to our cases, judging by the statements in his rather sketchy account. He regards stupor as being the most extreme degree of depressive retardation. [This possibility has been discussed in the chapter on Affect.] His description seems perhaps to include cases which we would regard as perplexity states or absorbed manias. Activity is reduced, they lie in bed mute, do not answer, may retract shyly at any approach, but on the other hand may not ward off pin pricks. Sometimes there is catalepsy and lack of will, again there may be aimless resistance to external interference. They hold anything put into their hands, turning it slowly as if ignorant of how to get rid of it. They may sit helpless before food or may allow spoon-feeding. Not rarely they are unclean. As to the mental content, he says they sometimes utter a few words, which give an insight into confused delusions that they are out of the world, that their brains are split, that they are talked about, or that something is going on in the lower part of the body. The affect is indefinite except for a certain bewilderment about their thoughts and an anxious uncertainty towards external interference. Intellectual processes suffer. They are disoriented and do not seem to understand the questions put to them. An answer "That is too complicated" may be made to some simple command. Kraepelin thinks that the disorder is sometimes more in the realm of the will than of thinking, for one patient could do a complicated calculation in the same time as a simple addition. After [273] recovery the memory for the period of the psychosis is poor and quite gone for parts of it. Occasionally there may be bursts of excitement, when they leave the bed; they may scold in a confused way or sing a popular song.

His manic stupor is a "mixed condition," a combination of retardation with elated mood. The condition is different from the depressive stupor in that activity is more frequent, either in constant fumbling with the bed clothes or in spasmodic scolding, joking, playing of pranks, assaultiveness, erotic behavior or decoration. The affect is usually apparent in surly expression or happy, or erotic, demeanor. They are usually fairly clear and oriented and often with good memory for the attack but with evasive explanations for their symptoms. One cannot make any classification of the ideas he quotes, but it is apparent from all his description that the minds of these "manic stupors" are not a blank but rather that there is a fairly full mental content.

Wernicke, unhampered by classifications of catatonia and manic-depressive insanity with inelastic boundaries, calls all stupor reactions akinetic psychoses with varying prognosis. He does not make Kraepelin's mistake of confusing the apathy of stupor with the retardation of depression, stating distinctly that the processes are different.

Bleuler also has grasped this discrimination. He points out that the thinking disorder in what he terms "Benommenheit" (dullness) differentiates such conditions from affectful depression with re [274] tardation. He writes, of course, mainly of dementia præcox, [28] but makes some remarks germane to our problem. In the first place he denies the existence of stupor as a clinical entity, except perhaps as the quintessence of "Benommenheit", it is the result of total blocking of mental processes. Consequently, he says, one can observe the external features of stupor in all akinetic catatonics, in marked depressive retardation, when there is a lack of interest, affect or will, in autism, with twilight states, as a result of negativism or, finally, when numerous hallucinations distract the patient's attention into a world of fancy. He notes that in all stupors (with the exception, perhaps, of "Benommenheit") the symptoms may disappear with appropriate psychic stimulation or that some reaction, no matter how larval, may be observed. He speaks, for instance, of the visits of relatives waking the patient up.

His only real group is "Benommenheit," which he separates out as a true clinical entity. This seems to correspond roughly with our "Partial Stupors." It is essentially an affectless, thinking disorder, usually acute, sometimes chronic, occurring among schizophrenics. He believes that it is the result of some organic process (intracranial pressure or toxin). Activity is much reduced or absent; they have poor understanding, answer slowly or confusedly; their actions are sometimes as ridiculous as those of people in panic (e.g., throwing a watch out [275] of the window when the house is on fire); the defect is best seen in writing, for large elisions are found in sentences. He was able to analyze only one case and she retained her affect; it was even labile and marked. One suspects that such a case might, perhaps, not really find a place in the "Benommenheit" group even as Bleuler himself describes it.

With the exception of Kirby, whose work has already been discussed in the introduction, we have been able to find only one author who has attempted any symptomatic discrimination of the recoverable and malignant catatonic states. Raecke [29] made a statistical study and found that 15.8% recovered, 10.8% improved, 54.4% remained in institutions, while 30% died. With the etiology mainly exogenous 20% recovered and 14.3% improved. A good outcome was seen in 30.2% of hereditary cases, while only 22.7% did well in the non-hereditary group. His most important contribution is in his formulation of good and bad symptoms. He thinks that dull, apathetic behavior with uncleanliness and loss of shame are not so unfavorable as has been thought. Malignant symptoms are grimacing with prolonged negativism but without essential affect anomaly, decided echopraxia and echolalia and protracted catalepsy. We would agree with this, although command automatisms have not been prominent either in our benign or malignant stupors.

[276]

Two writers have made special observations that should be confirmed and amplified before their significance can be established. Whitwell [30] thinks that in addition to a diminished activity of the heart there exists a pathological tension. Ziehen says that he also has frequently seen angiospastic pulse-curves in exhaustion stupor or acute dementia, but that other pulse pictures may be seen as well. Any such studies should be correlated rigorously with the clinical states before they can have any meaning. Wetzel [31] tested the psychogalvanic reflex in stupors and in normal persons who simulated stupors. He found them different.

Only one publication has come to our attention in which an attempt is made at psychological interpretation of various symptoms in stupor. Vogt [32] derives much from a restriction of the field of consciousness. Only one idea is present at a time, hence there is no inhibition and impulsiveness occurs. Similarly, if the idea appear from without, it, too, is not inhibited, which produces the suggestibility that in turn accounts for catalepsy. Stereotypy and perseveration are other evidences of this narrowness of thought content. Negativism is a state, he says, of perseverated muscular tension. [This would apply only to muscular rigidity.] So far as it [277] goes, this view seems sound. Of course it leaves the problem at that interesting point, Why the restriction of consciousness?

If stupor be a psychobiological reaction, it should occur, occasionally, in organic conditions just as the deliria of typhoid fever may contain many psychogenic elements. Gnauck [33] reports such a case. The patient, a woman, was poisoned by carbon dioxide. At first there was unconsciousness. Then, as she became clearer, it was apparent that she was clouded and confused. She soiled. Neurological symptoms were indefinite; enlargement of the left pupil, difficult gait and exaggerated tendon reflexes. Months later she was still apathetic, although her inactivity was sometimes interrupted by such silly acts as cutting up her shoes. After five months she recovered with only scattered memories of the early part of her psychosis. What seems like a typical stupor content was recalled, however. She thought she was standing in water and heard bells ringing.

Stupor-like reactions are not infrequent in connection with or following fevers. Bonhoeffer [34] describes a type that follows a febrile Daemmerzustand of a few hours or a day at most. The affect suddenly goes, disorientation sets in. Although outbreaks of anxiety may be intercurrent, the dominant picture is of stupor. Reactions are slowed, [278] often there is catalepsy. Sometimes there is a retention defect and confabulation to account for the recent past. Again the retention may be good. In the foreground stands a strong tendency to perseveration. This may affect speech to the point of an apparent aphasia or produce paragraphia. Plainly organic aphasia and focal neurological symptoms are sometimes seen.

As Knauer [35] has gone thoroughly into the question of the febrile stupors, the reader is referred to his paper for a digest of the literature on this topic. Mention has already been made in Chapter

IX to this publication, where the close resemblance of these rheumatic, to our benign functional, stupors has been noted. Discrimination seems to be possible only on the basis of delirium-like features being added in the organic group.

Footnotes:

[C] This chapter has been written mainly from material in Dr. Hoch's notes which was manifestly incomplete. No claim is made for its exhaustiveness.

The Editor.

[13] Dagonet, M. H.: "De la Stupeur dans les Maladies Mentales et de l'Affection mentale désignée sous le Nom de Stupidité." *Annales Medico-Psychologiques*, T. VII, 5e Serie, 1872.

[14] Newington, H. Hayes: "Some Observations on Different Forms of Stupor, and on Its Occurrence after Acute Mania in Females." *Journal of Mental Science*, Vol. XX, 1874, p. 372.

[15] Clouston: "Mental Diseases." J. & A. Churchill, 1904.

[16] Stern: "Ueber die akuten Situations-psychosen der Kriminellen." Abstracted, *Zeitschr. f. d. ges. Neurol. u. Psychiatrie*, Referate Bd. V, S. 554.

[17] Wilmanns, K.: "Statische Untersuchungen über Gefängnisspsychosen." *Allgemeine Zeitschr. f. Psychiatrie*, Bd. LXVII, S. 847.

[18] Kutner: "Ueber katatonischer Zustandsbilder bei Degenerierten." *Allgemeine Zeitschr. f. Psychiatrie*, Bd. LXVII, S. 375.

[19] Chotzen: "Fall von degenerativem Stupor." Abstracted, *Zeitschr. f. d. ges. Neur. u. Psychiatrie*, Referate, Bd. VI, S. 1077.

[20] Seelig: "Psychiatrischer Verein in Berlin, 1904." *Neurol. Centralbl.*, 1904, S. 421.

[21] Löwenstein: "Beitrag zur Differentialdiagnose des katatonische u. hysterische Stupors." *Allg. Zeitschr. f. Psychiatrie*, Bd. LXV.

[22] Gregor: "Über die Diagnose psychischer Prozesse im Stupor." Leipzig Meeting, 1907. Reported in *Neurol. Centralbl.*, 1907. S. 1083.

[23] Froederström: "La Dormeuse d'Okno. 32 ans de Stupeur, Guérison complète. Nouvelles Iconographies de la Salpétrière," 1912, No. 3. Reviewed by E. Bloch, *Neur. Centralbl.*, 1913, S. 852, and by Forster, *Zeitschr. f. d. ges. Neur. u. Psychiatrie*, Referate, Bd. VI, S. 510.

[24] Gadelius: "Ett ovanligt fall af stupor med nära 9-arig oafbruten tvangsmatning; uppvaknande; total amnesi; helsa" (*Hygiea*, 1894, LVI., Part 2, No. 10, p. 355). Abstracted by Walker Berger, *Neurol. Centralbl.*, 1895, S. 186.

[25] Leroy: "Un cas de stupeur, guéri au bout de deux ans et demi." *Bull. de la Soc. Clin. de Méd. Ment.*, III, 276, 1910. Abstracted in *Zeitschr. f. d. ges. Neurol. u. Psychiatrie*, Referate, Bd. II, S. 495.

[26] Myers, Charles S.: "Contributions to the Study of Shell Shock." *Lancet*, January 8, 1916, pp. 65-69. *Lancet*, September 6, 1916, pp. 461-467.

[27] Gucci, R.: "Sopra una particolarità del mutismo per stupore communicazione preventive." *Archivio italiano per le malattie nervose*, 1889, XXVI, 69-108. Reviewed in *Neurol. Centralbl.*, 1889, S. 659.

[28] "Dementia Præcox oder Gruppe der Schizophrenie" Aschaffenburg's "Handbuch der Psychiatrie."

[29] Raecke: "Zur Prognose der Katatonie." *Arch. f. Psychiatrie*, Bd. XLVII, 1, 1910.

[30] Whitwell: "A Study of the Pulse in Stupor." *Lancet*, Oct. 17, 1891. Reviewed by Ziehen, *Neurol. Centralbl.*, 1892, S. 290.

[31] Wetzel: "Die Diagnose von Stuporen." Baden-Baden Meeting of May, 1911. Reported in *Neurol. Centralbl.*, 1911, S. 886.

[32] Vogt, Ragner: "Zur Psychologie der Katatonischen Symptome." *Centralbl. für Nervenheilkunde*, 1902, S. 433.

[33] Gnauck, R.: "Stupor nach Kohlenoxydvergiftung" (*Charité-Annalen*, 1883, p. 409). Reviewed by Moeli, *Neurol. Centralbl.*, 1883, S. 237.

[34] Bonhoeffer: "Die Symptomatischen Psychosen," 1910.

[35] Knauer, A.: "Die im Gefolge des akuten Gelenkrheumatismus auftretenden psychischen Storungen." *Zeitschr. f. d. ges. Neurol. u. Psychiatrie*, Bd. XXI, S. 491-559.

[279]

INDEX

- absorption, 163
- activity, reduction of, 36, 100, 120
- acute dementia, 251
- adaptation, 107, 192
- adrenalin, 180
- affect, 9, 22, 32, 44, 113, 116, 117, *123*, 170
- affect, dissociation of, 128, 201, 205, 237
- affect, inappropriate, 216, 237
- affect, poverty of, 234
- affect, shallow, 127
- affectlessness, 171, 172
- affects, combination of, 245
- agitation, 156
- akinesis, 121
- akinetic psychoses, 4, 274
- albuminuria, 40
- allied to dementia præcox, 236, 260
- allied to manic-depressive, 236, 260
- allopsychic, 135
- ambivalence, 147
- amnesia, 9, 24, 68, 70, 267, 269
- anergic or unconscious stupor, 258
- anergic stupor, 255, 256
- anesthesia, 196, 212, 268
- anger, 118, 139
- angiospastic, 276
- animal, turning into, 171
- Antæus, 190
- apathy, 36, 48, 112, 122, 123, 151, 152, 163, 181, 195, 225, 237
- apathy, resemblance to absorption, 202
- anxiety, 122, 123, 126, 137, 153, 162, 166, 198, 226
- apoplexy, 224
- arteriosclerotic dementia, 80

- attention, 195
- atypical features, explanation of, 200
- autoerotism, 199
- automatism, 268

- Baillarger, 252
- behavior, 195
- "Benommenheit," 67, 273, 274
- bewilderment, 79, 112, 120, 126
- Bleuler, 67, 273
- blocking, 163
- blood-pressure, 181
- blushing, 9
- Bonhoeffer, 277
- boredom, 247
- bowels, interest in, 217
- brain tumor, 5
- breath, holding, 62
- Brierre de Boismont, 252
- burial, 111, 192

- Calculation, 23, 24
- Calvary, 111
- Cannon, 180
- Cases
    - Adele M. (Case 24), 220
    - Alice R., 135, 140, *192*
    - Anna G. (Case 1), *6* , 47, 48, 68, 74, 77, 109, 127, 136, 140, 145, 147, 183
    - Anna L. (Case 16), 135, *149* , 158
    - Anna M., 135
    - Annie K. (Case 5), 24 , 69, 72, 105, 110, 111, 136, 139, 141
    - [280] Bridget B., 135
    - Caroline de S. (Case 2), *11* , 68, 109, 141, 178, 193
    - Catherine H. (Case 23), *216*
    - Catherine M. (Case 18), *158*

- Catherine W. (Case 25), *221*
- Celia C. (Case 17), *155*
- Celia H. (Case 19), *167*
- Charles O., 143, 144, 178
- Charlotte W. (Case 12), *83*, 106, 112, 113, 116, 127, 136, 141, 144, 166, 201
- Emma K., 71, 140
- Harriett C., 138
- Helen M., 130
- Henrietta B., 138, 140
- Henrietta H. (Case 8), *42*, 74, 77, 105, 106, 110, 111, 115, 136
- Isabella M., 136, 144, 147
- Johanna B., 135, 138
- Johanna S. (Case 13), *91*, 120, 127, 136
- Josephine G., 138
- Laura A., 71, 77, 135, 138, 140, 142, 193
- Maggie H. (Case 14), 71, 96, 109, 140, 194
- Margaret C. (Case 10), *55*, 75, 78
- Mary C. (Case 7), *39*, 42, 71, 74, 77, 121, 136, 138, 178, 194
- Mary D. (Case 4), *20*, 47, 69, 70, 71, 74, 76, 109, 136, 145
- Mary F. (Case 3), *14*, 68, 105, 110, 111, 115, 140, 142, 164, 183
- Mary G., 140, 141
- Meta S. (Case 15), *99*, 109, 127, 135
- Nellie H. (Case 22), *214*
- Pearl F. (Case 9), *51*, 75, 142
- Rose S. (Case 21), *210*
- Rose Sch. (Case 6), *35*, 74, 75, 145
- Rosie K. (Case 11), *62*, 75, 105, 112, 178
- Winifred O'M. (Case 20), *207*
- catalepsy, 13, 21, 31, 32, 36, 86, 94, 95, 102, 115, 128, *143*, 144, 145, 147, 209, 211, 235, 239
- catatonia, 4, 5, 50, 128, 205, 236, 261
- catheterization, 85, 86, 102
- cemetery, 105, 112

- childbirth, 159
- childhood, 188, 195
- Chotzen, 262
- Christ, 86, 115
- Christian Science, 150
- circular psychosis, 5, 126
- circulation, 180
- Clark, 184
- clouding, 67
- Clouston, 258
- cocoon, 109
- coffin, 88, 106, 114
- coma, 176, 223
- concussion, aerial, 224
- confusion, 163
- constipation, 92
- convent, 117
- convulsive attacks, 15
- crime, 248
- crucifix, 88
- crucifixion, 86, 106, 114, 161
- crustaceans, 148
- cut-up idea, 94
- cyanosis, 32, 63, 180

- Dagonet, 3, 249, 250, 253, 254, 258
- death, feigned, 5, 83, 137, 196, 246
- death, mutual, 192
- death, projected, 198
- death, relation with affect, 110
- death ideas, 3, 46, 47, 50, 52, 58, 65, 83, 97, *104* , 107, 109, 110, 111, 114, 115, 119, 122, 136, 137, 138, 152, 153, 156, 159, 163, 166, 187, 190, 191, 192, 199, 212, 225, 235, 240
- death of others, 192
- deep stupor, *1* , 6, 41, 199
- deep stupor, explanation of, 197

- Delasiauve, 253
- [281] delirium, 176
- delusional stupor, 255, 256
- delusions, 165
- délire mélancholique, 252
- dementia præcox, 4, 5, 62, 123, 127, 128, 205, 225
- depression, 5, 117, 123, 137, 156, 236, 253
- depression, differentiation of, 48, 124, 226
- dermatographia, 102, 180
- deterioration, 210
- diabetes, 224
- diarrhea, 45, 64, 178
- dissociation, 225
- distress, 119, 122, 154, 156, 162
- dreams, 161, 190
- drooling, 132, 181
- drowning, 87, 192

- Earth, 107, 111, 190
- echolalia, 275
- echopraxia, 275
- ecstasy, 91, 162, 191
- *élan vital*, 123
- elation, 44, 91, 123, 127, 151, 157
- electric chair, 85, 110, 119
- electricity, 150
- emaciation, 8, 32, 58
- emotion, 62
- emotion, inconsistency of, 126
- emotions and contact with reality, 164
- energy, 187, 194
- epilepsy, 5, 183, 199, 224, 242, 254
- epileptic aura, 184
- epileptic confusion, 80
- epileptic deterioration, 80
- erotic, 161

- erotic ideas, 90
- Esquirol, 251
- Etoc-Demazy, 251
- Euripides, 2
- excretion, habits of, 230
- extroversion, 195

- family visits, 232
- father, 104, 109, 110
- fear, 111
- fever, 8, 13, 26, 32, 38, 40, 45, 64, 102, 160, *176*, 235, 241
- filthiness, 210
- fire, 151, 157
- flippancy, 129
- flushing, 27, 127, 128, 180
- food, refusal of, 99, 104
- Forel, 182
- Froederström, 265

- Gadelius, 267, 268
- Ganser reaction, 263
- Georget, 251
- German psychiatry, 259
- Gnauck, 277
- giggling, 206
- God, 115, 160, 162
- Golden Age, 187
- Gregor, 265
- Gucci, 271
- guilt, 157

- hair, loss of, 32, 58, 180
- heat production and loss, 179, 181, 242
- Heaven, 87, 88, 104, 106, 108, 109, 111, 114, 115, 117, 118, 160, 162, 166, 171, 191, 240
- Hell, 240

- Hoch, 164
- hyperæmia, 8
- hyperesthesia, 268
- hypochondria, 225, 253
- hypomania, 243
- hypnotism (see mesmerism), 145, 213
- hysteria, 3, 135, 184, 225, 264, 267, 269

- ideational content, 82, 235
- immobility, 85, 94, 196
- immorality, 150
- impulsiveness, 50, 113, 128, 172
- impurities in stupor reaction, 66
- inaccessibility, 141
- inactivity, 17, 30, 40, 48, 56, 62, 88, 97, 102, 123, *132* , 152, 163, 194, 225, 234, 238
- inactivity, patients' explanation of, 134
- incest ideas, 209
- [282] inconsistency of reaction, 134, 214, 215, 245
- incontinence (see *wetting* and *soiling*), 52, 57
- indifference, 123, 124, 142
- infantile reactions, 196
- infections, 5, *178* , 241
- insight, 157
- insomnia, 39
- instinct of self-preservation, 188, 191, 198
- interest, 99, 195
- internal secretions, 178
- internal thoughts, 163
- interruptions of stupor, 130, 197, 238, 244
- introversion, 164, 227
- involuntary nervous system, 178, 180
- involution melancholia, 129, 195, 225, 226

- jaundice, 21
- Jung, 107

- Kahlbaum, 4, 260
- Kirby, 4, 6, 164, 234
- Knauer, 175, 278
- Kraepelin, 4, 260, 269, 271, 272, 273
- Kutner, 262

- laughter, 56, 141
- Leroy, 269
- leucocytosis, 8, 13, 40, 64, 178
- levels, principle of, 198, 244
- Löwenstein, 264

- MacCurdy, 2, 184
- make-up, mental, 5
- malignant stupors, *205*
- mania (or manic), 5, 126, 137
- mania, absorbed, 125, 226, 245
- manic content, 166
- manic-depressive insanity, 149, 167
- manic-depressive insanity, mixed conditions in, 202
- manic-depressive insanity, pathology of, 174
- manic episodes, 191
- manic stupor, 125, 245, 253
- marriage, 160, 169
- masturbation, 196, 209, 219
- melancholic or conscious stupor, 258
- memory (see thinking disorder), 40, 67, 168, 195
- menstruation, 8, 56, 61, 100, 168, *182*, 236, 242
- mesmerism, 86, 114, 117, 141, 144
- Meyer, Adolf, 260
- Meyer, E., 261
- midday nap, 247
- mixed conditions, 202, 273
- Moeli, 264
- Moses, 108
- mother's body, 108

- movement, spontaneous, 133
- muscular resistiveness, 224
- mutism, 10, 22, 31, 57, 62, 88, 104, 124, 134, 209, 271
- mutual death, 165, 192, 196, 248
- Myers, 270, 271
- mystics, 3
- mythology, 107, 108, 190, 240

- negativism, 5, 31, 52, 56, 65, 128, *138* , 139, 199, 209, 225, 235, 238, 243, 276
- negativism, explanation of, 196
- nephritis, 224
- neuropsychic defect, 174
- neurotic, 150
- nervous, 159
- Newington, 3, 254, 255, 257
- Nirvana, 166, 188, 200, 248
- nourishment, 229, 242

- Œdipus, 165
- œstrous cycle, 182
- onset, 96
- onset, depressive, 99
- ophthalmic disease, 230
- Orestes, 2
- organic delirium, 175
- organic dementia, 67
- organic stupor, 223
- [283] orientation (see thinking disorder), 9, 53, 154, 156, 159, 170, 245
- Osiris, 108

- pain, 133
- Papanicolaou, 182
- paragraphia, 80
- paralysis, feeling of, 105

- paralysis, general, 5, 254
- partial stupor, *34*, 206
- perplexity, 125, 152, 153, 154, 155, 156, 160, 162, 164, 165, 169, 172, 208, 226, 245
- perplexity, differentiation of, 227
- perseveration, 145, 148, 276
- personality, 1
- perversity, 138
- physical disease, 175
- physical symptoms, *174*, 176
- Pinel, 249, 251
- poison, 97, 172
- primitive ideas, 108
- prison, 105, 169
- prognosis, 4, 5, *206*
- prostitution, 157, 161
- psychoanalysis, 161
- psychobiological reaction, 246
- psychogalvanic reflex, 276
- psychological explanation, 186
- psychological factors, 175
- pulse, 63, 92, 128, 180

- Rank, 107
- reality, 107, 187
- recuperation, 189
- rebirth, *107*, 110, 114, 115, 119, 120, 121, 122, 187, 189, 190, 191, 240
- regression, 187, 188, 191, 192, 194, 198, 199, 243
- religious visions or ideas, 2, 162
- resentment, 98
- resistiveness, 54, 97, 102, 112, 127, 129, 133, 141, 147, 156, 211, 225
- respiration, 180
- resurrection, 159
- restlessness, 53, 120, 169

- retention of urine, 224, 230
- rheumatism, 175
- rigidity, muscular, 142, 179
- Romberg sign, 262
- rousing, 176

- sadness, 111, 113, 121, 122, 124
- St. Catherine of Siena, 2
- St. Paul, 2
- saliva, 30, 63, 181
- scattered speech, 207, 208
- schizophrenia, 67, 214
- seclusiveness, 207
- secondary stupor, 259
- Seelig, 263
- self-injury, *50*, 57
- sexual excess, 251, 253, 258
- sexual ideas, 209, 219
- sexual sensations, 209
- ship, 87, 106, 118
- sick, 136
- skin, dry, 180
- skin, greasy, 43, 180
- sleep, 188, 189, 247
- slowing of thought, 125
- slowness, 85, 119, 160
- smearing of feces, 142
- smiling, 127
- social status, 236
- soiling, 30, 132, 172, 196, 225, 230, 235
- somatopsychic, 135
- sphincters, control of, 133
- spirits, 89
- spoiled child reaction, 129, 139
- starvation, 182
- stereotypy, 276

- Stern, 261
- stimulation, mental, 231, 246
- Stockard, 179, 182
- stubbornness, 142
- stupidity, 93
- stupor, diagnosis of, *223*
    - hysterical, 225
    - malignant, *205*, 206
    - organic, 223
    - reaction, *35*, 236
    - relation to manic-depressive insanity, 173
- sudden mental loss, 71
- suggestibility, 145, 198, 276
- [284] suicidal impulses, *50*, 84, 104, 116, 118, 128, 172, 230, 235, 240
- suicide, 188
- sulkiness, 129
- sullenness, 142
- suprarenals, 242
- swallowing, 133
- sweating, 63, 102, 179, 180
- swimming movements, 94
- syncopal attacks, 64

- tears, 95, 98, 117, 128, 153
- tense of ideas, 116
- thinking disorder, 22, 31, 37, 39, 41, 45, 48, 59, *67*, 75, 124, 125, 148, 152, 157, 235, 239, 247
- thinking disorder, explanation of, 195
- tongue, coated, 13
- toxins, 175
- trauma, 5, 224
- treatment, *229*

- ulceration of eyes, 133
- unconscious ideas, 163

- - motives, 186
- unconsciousness, physiological, 199, 224, 277
- underground, 240
- understanding, 67
- uneasiness, 93, 94, 95, 121
- unfaithfulness, 97
- unhappiness, 192
- urine, retention of, 31

- Villermay, 250
- Vogt, 276
- vomiting, 45

- water, 94, 95, 106, 107, 114, 120
- weakness, 137, 160
- wealth, 169
- wedding ring, 117
- weight (see emaciation), 38, 52, 61
- Wernicke, 3, 273
- wetting, 30, 40, 132, 151, 170, 172, 196, 225, 230, 235
- Wetzel, 276
- whining, 171, 225
- Whitwell, 276
- Wilmanns, 261
- womb, 108
- worry, 110
- writing, 27

- Ziehen, 276

www.ingramcontent.com/pod-product-compliance
Lightning Source LLC
Chambersburg PA
CBHW031614210526
45464CB00004B/1578